INSTANT VORTEX 2022

MOUTH-WATERING AND FRIENDLY-BUDGET RECIPES

SEAN DOUGLAS

Table of Contents

Applesauce and Chocolate Brownies

Prep time: 10 minutes | Cook time: 15 minutes | Serves 8

¼ cup unsweetened cocoa powder

¼ cup all-purpose flour

¼ teaspoon kosher salt

½ teaspoons baking powder

3 tablespoons unsalted butter, melted

½ cup granulated sugar

1 large egg

3 tablespoons unsweetened applesauce

¼ cup miniature semisweet chocolate chips

Coarse sea salt, to taste

1. Set the temperature of the air fryer oven to 300ºF (149ºC). Press Start to begin preheating.
2. In a large bowl, whisk together the cocoa powder, all-purpose flour, kosher salt, and baking powder.
3. In a separate large bowl, combine the butter, granulated sugar, egg, and applesauce, then use a spatula to fold in the cocoa powder mixture and the chocolate chips until well combined.
4. Spray a baking pan with nonstick cooking spray, then pour the mixture into the pan. Place the pan in the air

fryer oven and bake for 15 minutes or until a toothpick comes out clean when inserted in the middle.

5. Remove the brownies from the air fryer oven, sprinkle some coarse sea salt on top, and allow to cool in the pan on a wire rack for 20 minutes before cutting and serving.

Baked Apples

Prep time: 5 minutes | Cook time: 10 minutes | Serves 4

4 small apples, cored and cut in half

2 tablespoons salted butter or coconut oil, melted

2 tablespoons sugar

1 teaspoon apple pie spice

Ice cream, heavy cream, or whipped cream, for serving

1. Set the temperature of the air fryer oven to 350ºF (177ºC). Press Start to begin preheating.
2. Put the apples in a large bowl. Drizzle with the melted butter and sprinkle with the sugar and apple pie spice. Use the hands to toss, ensuring the apples are evenly coated.
3. Put the apples in the air fryer oven perforated pan and bake for 10 minutes. Pierce the apples with a fork to ensure they are tender.
4. Serve with ice cream, or top with a splash of heavy cream or a spoonful of whipped cream.

Banana and Walnut Cake

Prep time: 10 minutes | Cook time: 10 minutes | Serves 6

1 pound (454 g) bananas, mashed

8 ounces (227 g) flour

6 ounces (170 g) sugar

3.5 ounces (99 g) walnuts, chopped

2.5 ounces (71 g) butter

2 eggs

¼ teaspoon baking soda

1. Coat the inside of a baking dish with a little oil.
2. Set the temperature of the air fryer oven to 355ºF (179ºC). Press Start to begin preheating.
3. In a bowl combine the sugar, butter, egg, flour and soda using a whisk. Throw in the bananas and walnuts.
4. Transfer the mixture to the dish. Put the dish in the air fryer oven and bake for 10 minutes.
5. Reduce the temperature to 330ºF (166ºC) and bake for another 15 minutes. Serve hot.

Berry Crumble

Prep time: 10 minutes | Cook time: 15 minutes | Serves 4

For the Filling:

2 cups mixed berries

2 tablespoons sugar

1 tablespoon cornstarch

1 tablespoon fresh lemon juice

For the Toppin g :

¼ cup all-purpose flour

¼ cup rolled oats

1 tablespoon sugar

2 tablespoons cold unsalted butter, cut into small cubes

Whipped cream or ice cream (optional)

1. Set the temperature of the air fryer oven to 400ºF (204ºC). Press Start to begin preheating.
2. For the filling: In a round baking pan, gently mix the berries, sugar, cornstarch, and lemon juice until thoroughly combined.
3. For the topping: In a small bowl, combine the flour, oats, and sugar. Stir the butter into the flour mixture until the mixture has the consistency of bread crumbs.
4. Sprinkle the topping over the berries.
5. Put the pan in the air fryer oven and air fry for 15 minutes. Let cool for 5 minutes on a wire rack.
6. Serve topped with whipped cream or ice cream, if desired.

Black Forest Pies

Prep time: 10 minutes | Cook time: 15 minutes | Serves 6

3 tablespoons milk or dark chocolate chips

2 tablespoons thick, hot fudge sauce

2 tablespoons chopped dried cherries

1 (10-by-15-inch) sheet puff pastry, thawed

1 egg white, beaten

2 tablespoons sugar

½ teaspoon cinnamon

1. Set the temperature of the air fryer oven to 350ºF (177ºC). Press Start to begin preheating.
2. In a small bowl, combine the chocolate chips, fudge sauce, and dried cherries.
3. Roll out the puff pastry on a floured surface. Cut into 6 squares with a sharp knife.
4. Divide the chocolate chip mixture into the center of each puff pastry square. Fold the squares in half to make triangles. Firmly press the edges with the tines of a fork to seal.
5. Brush the triangles on all sides sparingly with the beaten egg white. Sprinkle the tops with sugar and cinnamon.
6. Put in the air fryer oven perforated pan and bake for 15 minutes or until the triangles are golden brown. The filling will be hot, so cool for at least 20 minutes before serving.

Bourbon Bread Pudding

Prep time: 10 minutes | Cook time: 20 minutes | Serves 4

3 slices whole grain bread, cubed

1 large egg

1 cup whole milk

2 tablespoons bourbon

½ teaspoons vanilla extract

¼ cup maple syrup, divided

½ teaspoons ground cinnamon

2 teaspoons sparkling sugar

1. Set the temperature of the air fryer oven to 270ºF (132ºC). Press Start to begin preheating.
2. Spray a baking pan with nonstick cooking spray, then place the bread cubes in the pan.
3. In a medium bowl, whisk together the egg, milk, bourbon, vanilla extract, 3 tablespoons of maple syrup, and cinnamon. Pour the egg mixture over the bread and press down with a spatula to coat all the bread, then sprinkle the sparkling sugar on top and bake for 20 minutes.
4. Remove the pudding from the air fryer oven and allow to cool in the pan on a wire rack for 10 minutes. Drizzle the remaining 1 tablespoon of maple syrup on top. Slice and serve warm.

Brazilian Pineapple Bake

Prep time: 5 minutes | Cook time: 16 minutes | Serves 4

½ cup brown sugar

2 teaspoons ground cinnamon

1 small pineapple, peeled, cored, and cut into spears

3 tablespoons unsalted butter, melted

1. Set the temperature of the air fryer oven to 400ºF (204ºC). Press Start to begin preheating.
2. In a small bowl, mix the brown sugar and cinnamon until thoroughly combined.
3. Brush the pineapple spears with the melted butter. Sprinkle the cinnamon-sugar over the spears, pressing lightly to ensure it adheres well.
4. Put the spears in the air fryer oven perforated pan in a single layer. (Depending on the size of the air fryer oven, you may have to do this in batches.) Bake for 10 minutes for the first batch (6 to 8 minutes for the next batch, as the air fryer oven will be preheated). Halfway through the cooking time, brush the spears with butter.
5. The pineapple spears are done when they are heated through and the sugar is bubbling. Serve hot.

Cardamom and Vanilla Custard

Prep time: 5 minutes | Cook time: 25 minutes | Serves 2

1 cup whole milk

1 large egg

2 tablespoons plus 1 teaspoon sugar

¼ teaspoon vanilla bean paste or pure vanilla extract

¼ teaspoon ground cardamom, plus more for sprinkling

1. Set the temperature of the air fryer oven to 350ºF (177ºC). Press Start to begin preheating.
2. In a medium bowl, beat together the milk, egg, sugar, vanilla, and cardamom.
3. Put two ramekins in the air fryer oven perforated pan. Divide the mixture between the ramekins. Sprinkle lightly with cardamom. Cover each ramekin tightly with aluminum foil. Bake for 25 minutes, or until a toothpick inserted in the center comes out clean.
4. Let the custards cool on a wire rack for 5 to 10 minutes.
5. Serve warm, or refrigerate until cold and serve chilled.

Chickpea Brownies

Prep time: 10 minutes | Cook time: 20 minutes | Serves 6

Vegetable oil

1 (15-ounce / 425-g) can chickpeas, drained and rinsed

4 large eggs

⅓ cup coconut oil, melted

⅓ cup honey

3 tablespoons unsweetened cocoa powder

1 tablespoon espresso powder (optional)

1 teaspoon baking powder

1 teaspoon baking soda

½ cup chocolate chips

1. Set the temperature of the air fryer oven to 325ºF (163ºC). Press Start to begin preheating.
2. Generously grease a baking pan with vegetable oil.
3. In a blender or food processor, combine the chickpeas, eggs, coconut oil, honey, cocoa powder, espresso powder (if using), baking powder, and baking soda. Blend or process until smooth. Transfer to the prepared pan and stir in the chocolate chips by hand.
4. Set the pan in the air fryer oven and bake for 20 minutes, or until a toothpick inserted into the center comes out clean.
5. Let cool in the pan on a wire rack for 30 minutes before cutting into squares.
6. Serve immediately.

Chocolate and Peanut Butter Lava Cupcakes

Prep time: 10 minutes | Cook time: 10 to 13 minutes | Serves 8

Nonstick baking spray with flour

1 1/3 cups chocolate cake mix

1 egg

1 egg yolk

¼ cup safflower oil

¼ cup hot water

1/3 cup sour cream

3 tablespoons peanut butter

1 tablespoon powdered sugar

1. Set the temperature of the air fryer oven to 350ºF (177ºC). Press Start to begin preheating.
2. Double up 16 foil muffin cups to make 8 cups. Spray each lightly with nonstick spray; set aside.
3. In a medium bowl, combine the cake mix, egg, egg yolk, safflower oil, water, and sour cream, and beat until combined.
4. In a small bowl, combine the peanut butter and powdered sugar and mix well. Form this mixture into 8 balls.
5. Spoon about ¼ cup of the chocolate batter into each muffin cup and top with a peanut butter ball. Spoon remaining batter on top of the peanut butter balls to cover them.
6. Arrange the cups in the air fryer oven perforated pan, leaving some space between each. Bake for 10 to 13 minutes or until the tops look dry and set.
7. Let the cupcakes cool for about 10 minutes, then serve warm.

Chocolate Cake

Prep time: 10 minutes | Cook time: 55 minutes | Serves 4

Unsalted butter, at room temperature

3 large eggs

1 cup almond flour

⅔ cup sugar

⅓ cup heavy cream

¼ cup coconut oil, melted

¼ cup unsweetened cocoa powder

1 teaspoon baking powder

¼ cup chopped walnuts

1. Set the temperature of the air fryer oven to 400ºF (204ºC). Press Start to begin preheating.
2. Generously butter a round baking pan. Line the bottom of the pan with parchment paper cut to fit.
3. In a large bowl, combine the eggs, almond flour, sugar, cream, coconut oil, cocoa powder, and baking powder. Beat with a hand mixer on medium speed until well blended and fluffy. (This will keep the cake from being too dense, as almond flour cakes can sometimes be.) Fold in the walnuts.
4. Pour the batter into the prepared pan. Cover the pan tightly with aluminum foil. Set the pan in the air fryer oven and bake for 45 minutes. Remove the foil and bake for 10 to 15 minutes more until a knife (do not use a toothpick) inserted into the center of the cake comes out clean.
5. Let the cake cool in the pan on a wire rack for 10 minutes. Remove the cake from the pan and let cool on the rack for 20 minutes before slicing and serving.

Chocolate Coconut Brownies

Prep time: 15 minutes | Cook time: 15 minutes | Serves 8

½ cup coconut oil

2 ounces (57 g) dark chocolate

1 cup sugar

2½ tablespoons water

4 whisked eggs

¼ teaspoon ground cinnamon

½ teaspoons ground anise star

¼ teaspoon coconut extract

½ teaspoons vanilla extract

1 tablespoon honey

½ cup flour

½ cup desiccated coconut

Sugar, for dusting

1. Set the temperature of the air fryer oven to 355ºF (179ºC). Press Start to begin preheating.
2. Melt the coconut oil and dark chocolate in the microwave.
3. Combine with the sugar, water, eggs, cinnamon, anise, coconut extract, vanilla, and honey in a large bowl.
4. Stir in the flour and desiccated coconut. Incorporate everything well.
5. Lightly grease a baking dish with butter. Transfer the mixture to the dish.
6. Put the dish in the air fryer oven and bake for 15 minutes.
7. Remove from the air fryer oven and allow to cool slightly.
8. Take care when taking it out of the baking dish. Slice it into squares.
9. Dust with sugar before serving.

Chocolate Croissants

Prep time: 5 minutes | Cook time: 24 minutes | Serves 8

1 sheet frozen puff pastry, thawed

⅓ cup chocolate-hazelnut spread

1 large egg, beaten

1. On a lightly floured surface, roll puff pastry into a 14-inch square. Cut pastry into quarters to form 4 squares. Cut each square diagonally to form 8 triangles.
2. Spread 2 teaspoons chocolate-hazelnut spread on each triangle; from wider end, roll up pastry. Brush egg on top of each roll.
3. Set the temperature of the air fryer oven to 375ºF (191ºC). Press Start to begin preheating. Air fry rolls in batches, 3 or 4 at a time, 8 minutes per batch, or until pastry is golden brown.
4. Cool on a wire rack; serve while warm or at room temperature.

Chocolate Molten Cake

Prep time: 5 minutes | Cook time: 10 minutes | Serves 4

3.5 ounces (99 g) butter, melted

3½ tablespoons sugar

3.5 ounces (99 g) chocolate, melted

1½ tablespoons flour

2 eggs

1. Set the temperature of the air fryer oven to 375ºF (191ºC). Press Start to begin preheating.
2. Grease four ramekins with a little butter.
3. Rigorously combine the eggs, butter, and sugar before stirring in the melted chocolate.
4. Slowly fold in the flour.
5. Spoon an equal amount of the mixture into each ramekin.
6. Put them in the air fryer oven and bake for 10 minutes
7. Put the ramekins upside-down on plates and let the cakes fall out. Serve hot.

Chocolate S'mores

Prep time: 5 minutes | Cook time: 3 minutes | Serves 12

12 whole cinnamon graham crackers

2 (1.55-ounce / 44-g) chocolate bars, broken into 12 pieces

12 marshmallows

1. Set the temperature of the air fryer oven to 350ºF (177ºC). Press Start to begin preheating.
2. Halve each graham cracker into 2 squares.
3. Put 6 graham cracker squares in the air fryer oven. Do not stack. Put a piece of chocolate into each. Bake for 2 minutes.
4. Open the air fryer oven and add a marshmallow onto each piece of melted chocolate. Bake for 1 additional minute.
5. Remove the cooked s'mores from the air fryer oven, then repeat steps 2 and 3 for the remaining 6 s'mores.
6. Top with the remaining graham cracker squares and serve.

Cinnamon Almonds

Prep time: 5 minutes | Cook time: 8 minutes | Serves 4

1 cup whole almonds

2 tablespoons salted butter, melted

1 tablespoon sugar

½ teaspoon ground cinnamon

1. Set the temperature of the air fryer oven to 300ºF (149ºC). Press Start to begin preheating.
2. In a medium bowl, combine the almonds, butter, sugar, and cinnamon. Mix well to ensure all the almonds are coated with the spiced butter.
3. Transfer the almonds to the air fryer oven perforated pan and shake so they are in a single layer. Bake for 8 minutes, stirring the almonds halfway through the cooking time.
4. Let cool completely before serving.

Cinnamon and Pecan Pie

Prep time: 10 minutes | Cook time: 25 minutes | Serves 4

1 pie dough

½ teaspoons cinnamon

¾ teaspoon vanilla extract

2 eggs

¾ cup maple syrup

⅛ teaspoon nutmeg

3 tablespoons melted butter, divided

2 tablespoons sugar

½ cup chopped pecans

1. Set the temperature of the air fryer oven to 370ºF (188ºC). Press Start to begin preheating.
2. In a small bowl, coat the pecans in 1 tablespoon of melted butter.
3. Transfer the pecans to the air fryer oven and allow them to toast for about 10 minutes.
4. Put the pie dough in a greased pie pan and add the pecans on top.
5. In a bowl, mix the rest of the ingredients. Pour this over the pecans.
6. Put the pan in the air fryer oven and bake for 25 minutes.
7. Serve immediately.

Curry Peaches, Pears, and Plums

Prep time: 5 minutes | Cook time: 5 minutes | Serves 6 to 8

2 peaches

2 firm pears

2 plums

2 tablespoons melted butter

1 tablespoon honey

2 to 3 teaspoons curry powder

1. Set the temperature of the air fryer oven to 325ºF (163ºC). Press Start to begin preheating.
2. Cut the peaches in half, remove the pits, and cut each half in half again. Cut the pears in half, core them, and remove the stem. Cut each half in half again. Do the same with the plums.
3. Spread a large sheet of heavy-duty foil on the work surface. Arrange the fruit on the foil and drizzle with the butter and honey. Sprinkle with the curry powder.
4. Wrap the fruit in the foil, making sure to leave some air space in the packet.
5. Put the foil package in the perforated pan and bake for 5 to 8 minutes, shaking the perforated pan once during the cooking time, until the fruit is soft.

1. Serve immediately.

Easy Almond Shortbread

Prep time: 5 minutes | Cook time: 12 minutes | Serves 8

½ cup (1 stick) unsalted butter

½ cup sugar

1 teaspoon pure almond extract

1 cup all-purpose flour

1. Set the temperature of the air fryer oven to 375ºF (191ºC). Press Start to begin preheating.
2. In a bowl of a stand mixer fitted with the paddle attachment, beat the butter and sugar on medium speed until fluffy, 3 to 4 minutes. Add the almond extract and beat until combined, about 30 seconds. Turn the mixer to low. Add the flour a little at a time and beat for about 2 minutes more until well incorporated.
3. Pat the dough into an even layer in a round baking pan. Put the pan in the air fryer oven and bake for 12 minutes.
4. Carefully remove the pan from air fryer oven. While the shortbread is still warm and soft, cut it into 8 wedges.
5. Let cool in the pan on a wire rack for 5 minutes. Remove the wedges from the pan and let cool on the rack before serving.

Easy Chocolate Donuts

Prep time: 5 minutes | Cook time: 8 minutes | Serves 8

1 (8-ounce / 227-g) can jumbo biscuits

Cooking oil

Chocolate sauce, for drizzling

1. Set the temperature of the air fryer oven to 375ºF (191ºC)
2. Separate the biscuit dough into 8 biscuits and place them on a flat work surface. Use a small circle cookie cutter or a biscuit cutter to cut a hole in the center of each biscuit. You can also cut the holes using a knife.
3. Spray the air fryer oven perforated pan with cooking oil.
4. Put 4 donuts in the air fryer oven. Do not stack. Spray with cooking oil. Air fry for 4 minutes.
5. Open the air fryer oven and flip the donuts. Air fry for an additional 4 minutes.
6. Remove the cooked donuts from the air fryer oven, then repeat steps 3 and 4 for the remaining 4 donuts.
7. Drizzle chocolate sauce over the donuts and enjoy while warm.

Lemony Apple Butter

Prep time: 10 minutes | Cook time: 1 hour | Makes 1¼ cups

Cooking spray

2 cups unsweetened applesauce

⅔ cup packed light brown sugar

3 tablespoons fresh lemon juice

½ teaspoon kosher salt

¼ teaspoon ground cinnamon

⅛ teaspoon ground allspice

1. Set the temperature of the air fryer oven to 340ºF (171ºC). Press Start to begin preheating.
2. Spray a metal cake pan with cooking spray. Whisk together all the ingredients in a bowl until smooth, then pour into the greased pan. Set the pan in the air fryer oven and bake until the apple mixture is caramelized, reduced to a thick purée, and fragrant, about 1 hour.
3. Remove the pan from the air fryer oven, stir to combine the caramelized bits at the edge with the rest, then let cool completely to thicken.
4. Serve immediately.

Fried Golden Bananas

Prep time: 5 minutes | Cook time: 7 minutes | Serves 6

1 large egg

¼ cup cornstarch

¼ cup plain bread crumbs

3 bananas, halved crosswise

Cooking oil

Chocolate sauce, for drizzling

1. Set the temperature of the air fryer oven to 350ºF (177ºC). Press Start to begin preheating.
2. In a small bowl, beat the egg. In another bowl, place the cornstarch. Put the bread crumbs in a third bowl.
3. Dip the bananas in the cornstarch, then the egg, and then the bread crumbs.
4. Spray the air fryer oven perforated pan with cooking oil.
5. Put the bananas in the perforated pan and spray them with cooking oil. Air fry for 5 minutes.
6. Open the air fryer oven and flip the bananas. Air fry for an additional 2 minutes.
7. Transfer the bananas to plates. Drizzle the chocolate sauce over the bananas, and serve.

Graham Cracker Cheesecake

Prep time: 10 minutes | Cook time: 20 minutes | Serves 8

1 cup graham cracker crumbs

3 tablespoons softened butter

1½ (8-ounce / 227-g) packages cream cheese, softened

$^{1}/_{3}$ cup sugar

2 eggs, beaten

1 tablespoon flour

1 teaspoon vanilla

¼ cup chocolate syrup

1. Set the temperature of the air fryer oven to 450ºF (232ºC). Press Start to begin preheating.
2. For the crust, combine the graham cracker crumbs and butter in a small bowl and mix well. Press into the bottom of a baking pan and put in the freezer to set.
3. For the filling, combine the cream cheese and sugar in a medium bowl and mix well. Beat in the eggs, one at a time. Add the flour and vanilla.
4. Remove $^2/_3$ cup of the filling to a small bowl and stir in the chocolate syrup until combined.
5. Pour the vanilla filling into the pan with the crust. Drop the chocolate filling over the vanilla filling by the spoonful. With a clean butter knife, stir the fillings in a zigzag pattern to marbleize them.
6. Bake for 20 minutes or until the cheesecake is just set.
7. Cool on a wire rack for 1 hour, then chill in the refrigerator until the cheesecake is firm.
8. Serve immediately.

Honey-Roasted Pears

Prep time: 5 minutes | Cook time: 20 minutes | Serves 4

2 large Bosc pears, halved and deseeded

3 tablespoons honey

1 tablespoon unsalted butter

½ teaspoon ground cinnamon

¼ cup walnuts, chopped

¼ cup part skim low-fat ricotta cheese, divided

1. Set the temperature of the air fryer oven to 350ºF (180ºC). Press Start to begin preheating.
2. In a baking pan, place the pears, cut-side up.
3. In a small microwave-safe bowl, melt the honey, butter, and cinnamon. Brush this mixture over the cut sides of the pears.
4. Pour 3 tablespoons of water around the pears in the pan. Roast the pears in the preheated air fryer oven for 20 minutes, or until tender when pierced with a fork and slightly crisp on the edges, basting once with the liquid in the pan.
5. Carefully remove the pears from the pan and place on a serving plate. Drizzle each with some liquid from the pan, sprinkle the walnuts on top, and serve with a spoonful of ricotta cheese.
6. Serve immediately.

Jelly Doughnuts

Prep time: 5 minutes | Cook time: 5 minutes | Serves 8

1 (16.3-ounce / 462-g) package large refrigerator biscuits

Cooking spray

1¼ cups good-quality raspberry jam

Confectioners' sugar, for dusting

1. Set the temperature of the air fryer oven to 350ºF (177ºC). Press Start to begin preheating.
2. Separate biscuits into 8 rounds. Spray both sides of rounds lightly with oil.
3. Spray the perforated pan with oil and place 3 to 4 rounds in the perforated pan. Air fry for 5 minutes, or until golden brown. Transfer to a wire rack; let cool. Repeat with the remaining rounds.
4. Fill a pastry bag, fitted with small plain tip, with raspberry jam; use tip to poke a small hole in the side of each doughnut, then fill the centers with the jam. Dust doughnuts with confectioners' sugar.
5. Serve immediately.

Lemony Blackberry Crisp

Prep time: 5 minutes | Cook time: 20 minutes | Serves 1

2 tablespoons lemon juice

$^{1}/_{3}$ cup powdered erythritol

¼ teaspoon xantham gum

2 cup blackberries

1 cup crunchy granola

1. Set the temperature of the air fryer oven to 350ºF (177ºC). Press Start to begin preheating.
2. In a bowl, combine the lemon juice, erythritol, xantham gum, and blackberries. Transfer to a round baking dish and cover with aluminum foil.
3. Put the dish in the air fryer oven and bake for 12 minutes.
4. Take care when removing the dish from the air fryer oven. Give the blackberries a stir and top with the granola.
5. Return the dish to the air fryer oven and bake for an additional 3 minutes, this time at 320ºF (160ºC). Serve once the granola has turned brown and enjoy.

Oatmeal and Carrot Cookie Cups

Prep time: 10 minutes | Cook time: 8 minutes | Makes 16 cups

3 tablespoons unsalted butter, at room temperature

¼ cup packed brown sugar

1 tablespoon honey

1 egg white

½ teaspoon vanilla extract

⅓ cup finely grated carrot

½ cup quick-cooking oatmeal

⅓ cup whole-wheat pastry flour

½ teaspoon baking soda

¼ cup dried cherries

1. Set the temperature of the air fryer oven to 350ºF (177ºC)
2. In a medium bowl, beat the butter, brown sugar, and honey until well combined.
3. Add the egg white, vanilla, and carrot. Beat to combine.
4. Stir in the oatmeal, pastry flour, and baking soda.
5. Stir in the dried cherries.
6. Double up 32 mini muffin foil cups to make 16 cups. Fill each with about 4 teaspoons of dough. Bake the cookie cups, 8 at a time, for 8 minutes, or until light golden brown and just set. Serve warm.

Oatmeal Raisin Bars

Prep time: 15 minutes | Cook time: 15 minutes | Serves 8

⅓ cup all-purpose flour

¼ teaspoon kosher salt

¼ teaspoon baking powder

¼ teaspoon ground cinnamon

¼ cup light brown sugar, lightly packed

¼ cup granulated sugar

½ cup canola oil

1 large egg

1 teaspoon vanilla extract

1⅓ cups quick-cooking oats

⅓ cup raisins

1. Set the temperature of the air fryer oven to 360ºF (182ºC). Press Start to begin preheating.
2. In a large bowl, combine the all-purpose flour, kosher salt, baking powder, ground cinnamon, light brown sugar, granulated sugar, canola oil, egg, vanilla extract, quick-cooking oats, and raisins.
3. Spray a baking pan with nonstick cooking spray, then pour the oat mixture into the pan and press down to evenly distribute. Place the pan in the air fryer oven and bake for 15 minutes or until golden brown.
4. Remove from the air fryer oven and allow to cool in the pan on a wire rack for 20 minutes before slicing and serving.

Orange Cake

Prep time: 10 minutes | Cook time: 23 minutes | Serves 8

Nonstick baking spray with flour

1¼ cups all-purpose flour

1/3 cup yellow cornmeal

¾ cup white sugar

1 teaspoon baking soda

¼ cup safflower oil

1¼ cups orange juice, divided

1 teaspoon vanilla

¼ cup powdered sugar

1. Set the temperature of the air fryer oven to 350ºF (177ºC). Press Start to begin preheating.
2. Spray a baking pan with nonstick spray and set aside.
3. In a medium bowl, combine the flour, cornmeal, sugar, baking soda, safflower oil, 1 cup of the orange juice, and vanilla, and mix well.
4. Pour the batter into the baking pan and place in the air fryer oven. Bake for 23 minutes or until a toothpick inserted in the center of the cake comes out clean.

5. Remove the cake from the oven and place on a cooling rack. Using a toothpick, make about 20 holes in the cake.
6. In a small bowl, combine remaining ¼ cup of orange juice and the powdered sugar and stir well. Drizzle this mixture over the hot cake slowly so the cake absorbs it.
7. Cool completely, then cut into wedges to serve.

Pear and Apple Crisp

Prep time: 10 minutes | Cook time: 20 minutes | Serves 6

½ pound (227 g) apples, cored and chopped

½ pound (227 g) pears, cored and chopped

1 cup flour

1 cup sugar

1 tablespoon butter

1 teaspoon ground cinnamon

¼ teaspoon ground cloves

1 teaspoon vanilla extract

¼ cup chopped walnuts

Whipped cream, for serving

1. Set the temperature of the air fryer oven to 340ºF (171ºC). Press Start to begin preheating.
2. Lightly grease a baking dish and place the apples and pears inside.
3. Combine the rest of the ingredients, minus the walnuts and the whipped cream, until a coarse, crumbly texture is achieved.
4. Pour the mixture over the fruits and spread it evenly. Top with the chopped walnuts.
5. Bake for 20 minutes or until the top turns golden brown.
6. When cooked through, serve at room temperature with whipped cream.

Pecan and Cherry Stuffed Apples

Prep time: 10 minutes | Cook time: 20 minutes | Serves 4

4 apples (about 1¼ pounds / 567 g)

¼ cup chopped pecans

⅓ cup dried tart cherries

1 tablespoon melted butter

3 tablespoons brown sugar

¼ teaspoon allspice

Pinch salt

Ice cream, for serving

1. Cut off top ½ inch from each apple; reserve tops. With a melon baller, core through stem ends without breaking through the bottom. (Do not trim bases.)
2. Set the temperature of the air fryer oven to 350ºF (177ºC). Press Start to begin preheating. Combine pecans, cherries, butter, brown sugar, allspice, and a pinch of salt. Stuff mixture into the hollow centers of the apples. Cover with apple tops. Put in the air fryer oven perforated pan, using tongs. Air fry for 20 to 25 minutes, or just until tender.
3. Serve warm with ice cream.

Pineapple and Chocolate Cake

Prep time: 10 minutes | Cook time: 35 to 40 minutes | Serves 4

2 cups flour

4 ounces (113 g) butter, melted

¼ cup sugar

½ pound (227 g) pineapple, chopped

½ cup pineapple juice

1 ounce (28 g) dark chocolate, grated

1 large egg

2 tablespoons skimmed milk

1. Set the temperature of the air fryer oven to 370ºF (188ºC). Press Start to begin preheating.
2. Grease a cake tin with a little oil or butter.
3. In a bowl, combine the butter and flour to create a crumbly consistency.
4. Add the sugar, chopped pineapple, juice, and grated dark chocolate and mix well.
5. In a separate bowl, combine the egg and milk. Add this mixture to the flour mixture and stir well until a soft dough forms.
6. Pour the mixture into the cake tin and transfer to the air fryer oven.
7. Bake for 35 to 40 minutes.
8. Serve immediately.

Pineapple Galette

Prep time: 10 minutes | Cook time: 40 minutes | Serves 2

¼ medium-size pineapple, peeled, cored, and cut crosswise into ¼-inch-thick slices

2 tablespoons dark rum

1 teaspoon vanilla extract

½ teaspoon kosher salt

Finely grated zest of ½ lime

1 store-bought sheet puff pastry, cut into an 8-inch round

3 tablespoons granulated sugar

2 tablespoons unsalted butter, cubed and chilled

Coconut ice cream, for serving

1. Set the temperature of the air fryer oven to 310ºF (154ºC). Press Start to begin preheating.
2. In a small bowl, combine the pineapple slices, rum, vanilla, salt, and lime zest and let stand for at least 10 minutes to allow the pineapple to soak in the rum.
3. Meanwhile, press the puff pastry round into the bottom and up the sides of a round metal cake pan and use the tines of a fork to dock the bottom and sides.
4. Arrange the pineapple slices on the bottom of the pastry in more or less a single layer, then sprinkle with the sugar and dot with the butter. Drizzle with the leftover juices from the bowl. Put the pan in the air fryer oven and bake until the pastry is puffed and golden brown and the pineapple is lightly caramelized on top, about 40 minutes.
5. Transfer the pan to a wire rack to cool for 15 minutes. Unmold the galette from the pan and serve warm with coconut ice cream.

Pumpkin Pudding

Prep time: 10 minutes | Cook time: 15 minutes | Serves 4

3 cups pumpkin purée

3 tablespoons honey

1 tablespoon ginger

1 tablespoon cinnamon

1 teaspoon clove

1 teaspoon nutmeg

1 cup full-fat cream

2 eggs

1 cup sugar

1. Set the temperature of the air fryer oven to 390ºF (199ºC). Press Start to begin preheating.
2. In a bowl, stir all the ingredients together to combine.
3. Grease the inside of a small baking dish.
4. Pour the mixture into the dish and transfer to the air fryer oven. Bake for 15 minutes. Serve warm.

Rich Chocolate Cookie

Prep time: 10 minutes | Cook time: 9 minutes | Serves 4

Nonstick baking spray with flour

3 tablespoons softened butter

$^1/_3$ cup plus 1 tablespoon brown sugar

1 egg yolk

½ cup flour

2 tablespoons ground white chocolate

¼ teaspoon baking soda

½ teaspoon vanilla

¾ cup chocolate chips

1. Set the temperature of the air fryer oven to 350ºF (177ºC). Press Start to begin preheating.
2. In a medium bowl, beat the butter and brown sugar together until fluffy. Stir in the egg yolk.
3. Add the flour, white chocolate, baking soda, and vanilla, and mix well. Stir in the chocolate chips.
4. Line a baking pan with parchment paper. Spray the parchment paper with nonstick baking spray with flour.
5. Spread the batter into the prepared pan, leaving a ½-inch border on all sides.
6. Bake for about 9 minutes or until the cookie is light brown and just barely set.
7. Remove the pan from the air fryer oven and let cool for 10 minutes. Remove the cookie from the pan, remove the parchment paper, and let cool on a wire rack.
8. Serve immediately.

Ricotta Lemon Poppy Seed Cake

Prep time: 15 minutes | Cook time: 55 minutes | Serves 4

Unsalted butter, at room temperature

1 cup almond flour

½ cup sugar

3 large eggs

¼ cup heavy cream

¼ cup full-fat ricotta cheese

¼ cup coconut oil, melted

2 tablespoons poppy seeds

1 teaspoon baking powder

1 teaspoon pure lemon extract

Grated zest and juice of 1 lemon, plus more zest for garnish

1. Set the temperature of the air fryer oven to 325ºF (163ºC). Press Start to begin preheating.
2. Generously butter a round baking pan. Line the bottom of the pan with parchment paper cut to fit.
3. In a large bowl, combine the almond flour, sugar, eggs, cream, ricotta, coconut oil, poppy seeds, baking powder, lemon extract, lemon zest, and lemon juice. Beat with a hand mixer on medium speed until well blended and fluffy.

4. Pour the batter into the prepared pan. Cover the pan tightly with aluminum foil. Set the pan in the air fryer oven and bake for 45 minutes. Remove the foil and bake for 10 to 15 minutes more until a knife (do not use a toothpick) inserted into the center of the cake comes out clean.
5. Let the cake cool in the pan on a wire rack for 10 minutes. Remove the cake from pan and let it cool on the rack for 15 minutes before slicing.
6. Top with additional lemon zest, slice and serve.

Simple Apple Turnovers

Prep time: 10 minutes | Cook time: 10 minutes | Serves 4

1 apple, peeled, quartered, and thinly sliced

½ teaspoons pumpkin pie spice

Juice of ½ lemon

1 tablespoon granulated sugar

Pinch of kosher salt

6 sheets phyllo dough

1. Set the temperature of the air fryer oven to 330ºF (166ºC). Press Start to begin preheating.
2. In a medium bowl, combine the apple, pumpkin pie spice, lemon juice, granulated sugar, and kosher salt.
3. Cut the phyllo dough sheets into 4 equal pieces and place individual tablespoons of apple filling in the center of each piece, then fold in both sides and roll from front to back.
4. Spray the air fryer oven perforated pan with nonstick cooking spray, then place the turnovers in the perforated pan and bake for 10 minutes or until golden brown.
5. Remove the turnovers from the air fryer oven and allow to cool on a wire rack for 10 minutes before serving.

Simple Pineapple Sticks

Prep time: 5 minutes | Cook time: 10 minutes | Serves 4

½ fresh pineapple, cut into sticks

¼ cup desiccated coconut

1. Set the temperature of the air fryer oven to 400ºF (204ºC). Press Start to begin preheating.
2. Coat the pineapple sticks in the desiccated coconut and put each one in the air fryer oven perforated pan.
3. Air fry for 10 minutes.
4. Serve immediately

Spice Cookies

Prep time: 15 minutes | Cook time: 12 minutes | Serves 4

4 tablespoons (½ stick) unsalted butter, at room temperature

2 tablespoons agave nectar

1 large egg

2 tablespoons water

2½ cups almond flour

½ cup sugar

2 teaspoons ground ginger

1 teaspoon ground cinnamon

½ teaspoon freshly grated nutmeg

1 teaspoon baking soda

¼ teaspoon kosher salt

1. Set the temperature of the air fryer oven to 325ºF (163ºC). Press Start to begin preheating.
2. Line the bottom of the air fryer oven perforated pan with parchment paper cut to fit.
3. In a large bowl using a hand mixer, beat together the butter, agave, egg, and water on medium speed until fluffy.

4. Add the almond flour, sugar, ginger, cinnamon, nutmeg, baking soda, and salt. Beat on low speed until well combined.
5. Roll the dough into 2-tablespoon balls and arrange them on the parchment paper in the perforated pan. Bake for 12 minutes, or until the tops of cookies are lightly browned.
6. Transfer to a wire rack and let cool completely.
7. Serve immediately

Air Fried Baby Back Ribs

Prep time: 5 minutes | Cook time: 30 minutes | Serves 2

2 teaspoons red pepper flakes

¾ ground ginger

3 cloves minced garlic

Salt and ground black pepper, to taste

2 baby back ribs

1. Set the temperature of the air fryer oven to 350ºF (177ºC). Press Start to begin preheating.
2. Combine the red pepper flakes, ginger, garlic, salt and pepper in a bowl, making sure to mix well. Massage the mixture into the baby back ribs.
3. Air fry the ribs in the air fryer oven for 30 minutes.
4. Take care when taking the rubs out of the air fryer oven. Put them on a serving dish and serve.

Air Fried Beef Ribs

Prep time: 20 minutes | Cook time: 8 minutes | Serves 4

1 pound (454 g) meaty beef ribs, rinsed and drained

3 tablespoons apple cider vinegar

1 cup coriander, finely chopped

1 tablespoon fresh basil leaves, chopped

2 garlic cloves, finely chopped

1 chipotle powder

1 teaspoon fennel seeds

1 teaspoon hot paprika

Kosher salt and black pepper, to taste

½ cup vegetable oil

1. Coat the ribs with the remaining ingredients and refrigerate for at least 3 hours.
2. Set the temperature of the air fryer oven to 360ºF (182ºC). Press Start to begin preheating.
3. Separate the ribs from the marinade and put them on a grill pan. Air fry for 8 minutes.
4. Pour the remaining marinade over the ribs before serving.

Air Fried Lamb Ribs

Prep time: 5 minutes | Cook time: 18 minutes | Serves 4

2 tablespoons mustard

1 pound (454 g) lamb ribs

1 teaspoon rosemary, chopped

Salt and ground black pepper, to taste

¼ cup mint leaves, chopped

1 cup Green yogurt

1. Set the temperature of the air fryer oven to 350ºF (177ºC). Press Start to begin preheating.
2. Use a brush to apply the mustard to the lamb ribs, and season with rosemary, salt, and pepper.
3. Air fry the ribs in the air fryer oven for 18 minutes.
4. Meanwhile, combine the mint leaves and yogurt in a bowl.
5. Remove the lamb ribs from the air fryer oven when cooked and serve with the mint yogurt.

Air Fried London Broil

Prep time: 15 minutes | Cook time: 25 minutes | Serves 8

2 pounds (907 g) London broil

3 large garlic cloves, minced

3 tablespoons balsamic vinegar

3 tablespoons whole-grain mustard

2 tablespoons olive oil

Sea salt and ground black pepper, to taste

½ teaspoons dried hot red pepper flakes

1. Wash and dry the London broil. Score its sides with a knife.
2. Mix the remaining ingredients. Rub this mixture into the broil, coating it well. Allow to marinate for a minimum of 3 hours.
3. Set the temperature of the air fryer oven to 400ºF (204ºC). Press Start to begin preheating.
4. Air fry the meat for 15 minutes. Turn it over and air fry for an additional 10 minutes before serving.

Air Fried Ribeye Steak

Prep time: 5 minutes | Cook time: 15 minutes | Serves 1

1 (1-pound / 454-g) ribeye steak

Salt and ground black pepper, to taste

1 tablespoon peanut oil

½ tablespoon butter

½ teaspoon thyme, chopped

1. Set the temperature of the air fryer oven to 400ºF (204ºC). Press Start to begin preheating.
2. Season the steaks with salt and pepper.
3. Grease a skillet with peanut oil. Sear the steak over medium heat for 2 minutes.
4. Turn over the steak and place in the air fryer oven for 6 minutes.
5. Take out the steak from the air fryer oven and place it back on the stove top on low heat to keep warm.
6. Toss in the butter and thyme and air fry for 3 minutes.
7. Rest for 5 minutes and serve.

Avocado Buttered Flank Steak

Prep time: 5 minutes | Cook time: 12 minutes | Serves 1

1 flank steak

Salt and ground black pepper, to taste

2 avocados

2 tablespoons butter, melted

½ cup chimichurri sauce

1. Rub the flank steak with salt and pepper to taste and leave to sit for 20 minutes.
2. Set the temperature of the air fryer oven to 400ºF (204ºC) and place a rack inside.
3. Halve the avocados and take out the pits. Spoon the flesh into a bowl and mash with a fork. Mix in the melted butter and chimichurri sauce, making sure everything is well combined.
4. Put the steak in the air fryer oven and air fry for 6 minutes. Flip over and allow to air fry for another 6 minutes.
5. Serve the steak with the avocado butter.

Bacon and Pear Stuffed Pork Chops

Prep time: 20 minutes | Cook time: 24 minutes | Serves 3

4 slices bacon, chopped

1 tablespoon butter

½ cup finely diced onion

⅓ cup chicken stock

1½ cups seasoned stuffing cubes

1 egg, beaten

½ teaspoon dried thyme

½ teaspoon salt

⅛ teaspoon freshly ground black pepper

1 pear, finely diced

⅓ cup crumbled blue cheese

3 boneless center-cut pork chops (2-inch thick)

Olive oil, for greasing

Salt and freshly ground black pepper, to taste

1. Set the temperature of the air fryer oven to 400ºF (204ºC). Press Start to begin preheating.
2. Put the bacon into the air fryer oven perforated pan and air fry for 6 minutes, stirring halfway through the cooking time. Remove the bacon and set it aside on a

paper towel. Pour out the grease from the bottom of the air fryer oven.

3. To make the stuffing, melt the butter in a medium saucepan over medium heat on the stovetop. Add the onion and sauté for a few minutes until it starts to soften. Add the chicken stock and simmer for 1 minute. Remove the pan from the heat and add the stuffing cubes. Stir until the stock has been absorbed. Add the egg, dried thyme, salt and freshly ground black pepper, and stir until combined. Fold in the diced pear and crumbled blue cheese.
4. Put the pork chops on a cutting board. Using the palm of the hand to hold the chop flat and steady, slice into the side of the pork chop to make a pocket in the center of the chop. Leave about an inch of chop uncut and make sure you don't cut all the way through the pork chop. Brush both sides of the pork chops with olive oil and season with salt and freshly ground black pepper. Stuff each pork chop with a third of the stuffing, packing the stuffing tightly inside the pocket.
5. Set the temperature of the air fryer oven to 360ºF (182ºC). Press Start to begin preheating.
6. Spray or brush the sides of the air fryer oven perforated pan with oil. Put the pork chops in the perforated pan

with the open, stuffed edge of the pork chop facing the outside edges of the perforated pan.

7. Air fry the pork chops for 18 minutes, turning the pork chops over halfway through the cooking time. When the chops are done, let them rest for 5 minutes and then transfer to a serving platter.

Bacon Wrapped Pork with Apple Gravy

Prep time: 10 minutes | Cook time: 25 minutes | Serves 4

Pork:

1 tablespoons Dijon mustard

1 pork tenderloin

3 strips bacon

Apple Gravy:

3 tablespoons ghee, divided

1 shallot, chopped

2 apples

1 tablespoon almond flour

1 cup vegetable broth

½ teaspoon Dijon mustard

1. Set the temperature of the air fryer oven to 360ºF (182ºC). Press Start to begin preheating.
2. Spread Dijon mustard all over tenderloin and wrap meat with strips of bacon.
3. Put into air fryer oven and air fry for 12 minutes. Use a meat thermometer to check for doneness.
4. To make sauce, heat 1 tablespoon of ghee in a pan and add shallots. Cook for 1 minute.
5. Then add apples, cooking for 4 minutes until softened.

6. Add flour and 2 tablespoons of ghee to make a roux. Add broth and mustard, stirring well to combine.
7. When sauce starts to bubble, add 1 cup of sautéed apples, cooking until sauce thickens.
8. Once pork tenderloin is cooked, allow to sit 8 minutes to rest before slicing.
9. Serve topped with apple gravy.

Barbecue Pork Ribs

Prep time: 5 minutes | Cook time: 30 minutes | Serves 4

1 tablespoon barbecue dry rub

1 teaspoon mustard

1 tablespoon apple cider vinegar

1 teaspoon sesame oil

1 pound (454 g) pork ribs, chopped

1. Combine the dry rub, mustard, apple cider vinegar, and sesame oil, then coat the ribs with this mixture. Refrigerate the ribs for 20 minutes.
2. Set the temperature of the air fryer oven to 360ºF (182ºC). Press Start to begin preheating.
3. When the ribs are ready, place them in the air fryer oven and air fry for 15 minutes. Flip them and air fry on the other side for a further 15 minutes.
4. Serve immediately.

BBQ Pork Steaks

Prep time: 5 minutes | Cook time: 15 minutes | Serves 4

4 pork steaks

1 tablespoon Cajun seasoning

2 tablespoons BBQ sauce

1 tablespoon vinegar

1 teaspoon soy sauce

½ cup brown sugar

½ cup ketchup

1. Set the temperature of the air fryer oven to 290ºF (143ºC). Press Start to begin preheating.
2. Sprinkle pork steaks with Cajun seasoning.
3. Combine remaining ingredients and brush onto steaks.
4. Add coated steaks to air fryer oven. Air fry 15 minutes until just browned.
5. Serve immediately.

Beef and Cheddar Burgers

Prep time: 20 minutes | Cook time: 25 minutes | Serves 4

1 tablespoon olive oil

1 onion, sliced into rings

1 teaspoon garlic, minced or puréed

1 teaspoon mustard

1 teaspoon basil

1 teaspoon mixed herbs

Salt and ground black pepper, to taste

1 teaspoon tomato, puréed

4 buns

1 ounce (28 g) Cheddar cheese

10.5 ounces (298 g) beef, minced

Salad leaves

1. Set the temperature of the air fryer oven to 390ºF (199ºC). Press Start to begin preheating.
2. Grease the air fryer oven with olive oil and allow it to warm up.
3. Put the diced onion in the air fryer oven and air fry until they turn golden brown.
4. Mix the garlic, mustard, basil, herbs, salt, and pepper, and air fry for 25 minutes.

5. Lay 2 to 3 onion rings and puréed tomato on two of the buns. Put one slice of cheese and the layer of beef on top. Top with salad leaves and any other condiments you desire before closing off the sandwich with the other buns.
6. Serve immediately.

Beef and Pork Sausage Meatloaf

Prep time: 20 minutes | Cook time: 25 minutes | Serves 4

¾ pound (340 g) ground chuck

4 ounces (113 g) ground pork sausage

1 cup shallots, finely chopped

2 eggs, well beaten

3 tablespoons plain milk

1 tablespoon oyster sauce

1 teaspoon porcini mushrooms

½ teaspoon cumin powder

1 teaspoon garlic paste

1 tablespoon fresh parsley

Salt and crushed red pepper flakes, to taste

1 cup crushed saltines

Cooking spray

1. Set the temperature of the air fryer oven to 360ºF (182ºC). Press Start to begin preheating. Spritz a baking dish with cooking spray.
2. Mix all the ingredients in a large bowl, combining everything well.
3. Transfer to the baking dish and bake in the air fryer oven for 25 minutes.
4. Serve hot.

Beef and Spinach Rolls

Prep time: 10 minutes | Cook time: 14 minutes | Serves 2

3 teaspoons pesto

2 pounds (907 g) beef flank steak

6 slices provolone cheese

3 ounces (85 g) roasted red bell peppers

¾ cup baby spinach

1 teaspoon sea salt

1 teaspoon black pepper

1. Set the temperature of the air fryer oven to 400ºF (204ºC). Press Start to begin preheating.
2. Spoon equal amounts of the pesto onto each flank steak and spread it across evenly.
3. Put the cheese, roasted red peppers and spinach on top of the meat, about three-quarters of the way down.
4. Roll the steak up, holding it in place with toothpicks. Sprinkle with the sea salt and pepper.
5. Put inside the air fryer oven and air fry for 14 minutes, turning halfway through the cooking time.
6. Allow the beef to rest for 10 minutes before slicing up and serving.

Beef and Vegetable Cubes

Prep time: 15 minutes | Cook time: 17 minutes | Serves 4

2 tablespoons olive oil

1 tablespoon apple cider vinegar

1 teaspoon fine sea salt

½ teaspoons ground black pepper

1 teaspoon shallot powder

¾ teaspoon smoked cayenne pepper

½ teaspoons garlic powder

¼ teaspoon ground cumin

1 pound (454 g) top round steak, cut into cubes

4 ounces (113 g) broccoli, cut into florets

4 ounces (113 g) mushrooms, sliced

1 teaspoon dried basil

1 teaspoon celery seeds

1. Massage the olive oil, vinegar, salt, black pepper, shallot powder, cayenne pepper, garlic powder, and cumin into the cubed steak, ensuring to coat each piece evenly.
2. Allow to marinate for a minimum of 3 hours.
3. Set the temperature of the air fryer oven to 365ºF (185ºC). Press Start to begin preheating.

4. Put the beef cubes in the air fryer oven perforated pan and air fry for 12 minutes.
5. When the steak is cooked through, place it in a bowl.
6. Wipe the grease from the perforated pan and pour in the vegetables. Season them with basil and celery seeds.
7. Increase the temperature of the air fryer oven to 400ºF (204ºC) and air fry for 5 to 6 minutes. When the vegetables are hot, serve them with the steak.

Beef Cheeseburger Egg Rolls

Prep time: 15 minutes | Cook time: 8 minutes | Makes 6 egg rolls

8 ounces (227 g) raw lean ground beef

½ cup chopped onion

½ cup chopped bell pepper

¼ teaspoon onion powder

¼ teaspoon garlic powder

3 tablespoons cream cheese

1 tablespoon yellow mustard

3 tablespoons shredded Cheddar cheese

6 chopped dill pickle chips

6 egg roll wrappers

1. Set the temperature of the air fryer oven to 392ºF (200ºC). Press Start to begin preheating.
2. In a skillet, add the beef, onion, bell pepper, onion powder, and garlic powder. Stir and crumble beef until fully cooked, and vegetables are soft.
3. Take skillet off the heat and add cream cheese, mustard, and Cheddar cheese, stirring until melted.
4. Pour beef mixture into a bowl and fold in pickles.

5. Lay out egg wrappers and divide the beef mixture into each one. Moisten egg roll wrapper edges with water. Fold sides to the middle and seal with water.
6. Repeat with all other egg rolls.
7. Put rolls into air fryer oven, one batch at a time. Air fry for 8 minutes.
8. Serve immediately.

Beef Chuck Cheeseburgers

Prep time: 10 minutes | Cook time: 15 minutes | Serves 4

¾ pound (340 g) ground beef chuck

1 envelope onion soup mix

Kosher salt and freshly ground black pepper, to taste

1 teaspoon paprika

4 slices Monterey Jack cheese

4 ciabatta rolls

1. In a bowl, stir together the ground chuck, onion soup mix, salt, black pepper, and paprika to combine well.
2. Set the temperature of the air fryer oven to 385ºF (196ºC). Press Start to begin preheating.
3. Take four equal portions of the mixture and mold each one into a patty. Transfer to the air fryer oven and air fry for 10 minutes.
4. Put the slices of cheese on the top of the burgers.
5. Air fry for another minute before serving on ciabatta rolls.

Beef Chuck with Brussels Sprouts

Prep time: 20 minutes | Cook time: 15 minutes | Serves 4

1 pound (454 g) beef chuck shoulder steak

2 tablespoons vegetable oil

1 tablespoon red wine vinegar

1 teaspoon fine sea salt

½ teaspoon ground black pepper

1 teaspoon smoked paprika

1 teaspoon onion powder

½ teaspoon garlic powder

½ pound (227 g) Brussels sprouts, cleaned and halved

½ teaspoon fennel seeds

1 teaspoon dried basil

1 teaspoon dried sage

1. Massage the beef with the vegetable oil, wine vinegar, salt, black pepper, paprika, onion powder, and garlic powder, coating it well.
2. Allow to marinate for a minimum of 3 hours.
3. Set the temperature of the air fryer oven to 390ºF (199ºC). Press Start to begin preheating.

4. Remove the beef from the marinade and put in the preheated air fryer oven. Air fry for 10 minutes. Flip the beef halfway through.
5. Put the prepared Brussels sprouts in the air fryer oven along with the fennel seeds, basil, and sage.
6. Lower the heat to 380ºF (193ºC) and air fry everything for another 5 minutes.
7. Give them a good stir. Air fry for an additional 10 minutes.
8. Serve immediately.

Beef Egg Rolls

Prep time: 15 minutes | Cook time: 12 minutes | Makes 8 egg rolls

½ chopped onion

2 garlic cloves, chopped

½ packet taco seasoning

Salt and ground black pepper, to taste

1 pound (454 g) lean ground beef

½ can cilantro lime rotel

16 egg roll wrappers

1 cup shredded Mexican cheese

1 tablespoon olive oil

1 teaspoon cilantro

1. Set the temperature of the air fryer oven to 400ºF (205ºC). Press Start to begin preheating.
2. Add onions and garlic to a skillet, cooking until fragrant. Then add taco seasoning, pepper, salt, and beef, cooking until beef is broke up into tiny pieces and cooked thoroughly.
3. Add rotel and stir well.
4. Lay out egg wrappers and brush with a touch of water to soften a bit.
5. Load wrappers with beef filling and add cheese to each.
6. Fold diagonally to close and use water to secure edges.
7. Brush filled egg wrappers with olive oil and add to the air fryer oven.
8. Air fry 8 minutes, flip, and air fry for another 4 minutes.
9. Serve sprinkled with cilantro.

Beef Loin with Thyme and Parsley

Prep time: 5 minutes | Cook time: 15 minutes | Serves 4

1 tablespoon butter, melted

¼ dried thyme

1 teaspoon garlic salt

¼ teaspoon dried parsley

1 pound (454 g) beef loin

1. In a bowl, combine the melted butter, thyme, garlic salt, and parsley.
2. Cut the beef loin into slices and generously apply the seasoned butter using a brush.
3. Set the temperature of the air fryer oven to 400ºF (204ºC) and place a rack inside.
4. Air fry the beef on the rack for 15 minutes.
5. Take care when removing it and serve hot.

Beef Steak Fingers

Prep time: 5 minutes | Cook time: 8 minutes | Serves 4

4 small beef cube steaks

Salt and ground black pepper, to taste

½ cup flour

Cooking spray

1. Set the temperature of the air fryer oven to 390ºF (199ºC). Press Start to begin preheating.
2. Cut cube steaks into 1-inch-wide strips.
3. Sprinkle lightly with salt and pepper to taste.
4. Roll in flour to coat all sides.
5. Spritz air fryer oven perforated pan with cooking spray.
6. Put steak strips in air fryer oven perforated pan in a single layer. Spritz top of steak strips with oil or cooking spray.
7. Air fry for 4 minutes, turn strips over, and spritz with cooking spray.
8. Air fry 4 more minutes and test with fork for doneness. Steak fingers should be crispy outside with no red juices inside.
9. Repeat steps 5 through 7 to air fry remaining strips.
10. Serve immediately.

Carne Asada Tacos

Prep time: 5 minutes | Cook time: 14 minutes | Serves 4

$^{1}/_{3}$ cup olive oil

1½ pounds (680 g) flank steak

Salt and freshly ground black pepper, to taste

⅓ cup freshly squeezed lime juice

½ cup chopped fresh cilantro

4 teaspoons minced garlic

1 teaspoon ground cumin

1 teaspoon chili powder

1. Brush the air fryer oven perforated pan with olive oil.
2. Put the flank steak in a large mixing bowl. Season with salt and pepper.
3. Add the lime juice, cilantro, garlic, cumin, and chili powder and toss to coat the steak.
4. For the best flavor, let the steak marinate in the refrigerator for about 1 hour.
5. Set the temperature of the air fryer oven to 400ºF (204ºC)
6. Put the steak in the air fryer oven perforated pan. Air fry for 7 minutes. Flip the steak. Air fry for 7 minutes more

or until an internal temperature reaches at least 145ºF (63ºC).

7. Let the steak rest for about 5 minutes, then cut into strips to serve.

Char Siew

Prep time: 10 minutes | Cook time: 20 minutes | Serves 4 to 6

1 strip of pork shoulder butt with a good amount of fat marbling

Olive oil, for brushing the pan

Marinade:

1 teaspoon sesame oil

4 tablespoons raw honey

1 teaspoon low-sodium dark soy sauce

1 teaspoon light soy sauce

1 tablespoon rose wine

2 tablespoons Hoisin sauce

1. Combine the marinade ingredients together in a Ziploc bag. Put pork in bag, making sure all sections of pork strip are engulfed in the marinade. Chill for at least 3 hours.
2. Take out the strip 30 minutes before planning to roast and set the temperature of the air fryer oven to 350ºF (177ºC). Press Start to begin preheating.
3. Put foil on small pan and brush with olive oil. Put marinated pork strip onto prepared pan.
4. Roast in the air fryer oven for 20 minutes.
5. Glaze with marinade every 5 to 10 minutes.
6. Remove strip and leave to cool a few minutes before slicing.
7. Serve immediately.

Cheddar Bacon Burst with Spinach

Prep time: 5 minutes | Cook time: 60 minutes | Serves 8

30 slices bacon

1 tablespoon Chipotle seasoning

2 teaspoons Italian seasoning

2½ cups Cheddar cheese

4 cups raw spinach

1. Set the temperature of the air fryer oven to 375ºF (191ºC). Press Start to begin preheating.
2. Weave the bacon into 15 vertical pieces and 12 horizontal pieces. Cut the extra 3 in half to fill in the rest, horizontally.
3. Season the bacon with Chipotle seasoning and Italian seasoning.
4. Add the cheese to the bacon.
5. Add the spinach and press down to compress.
6. Tightly roll up the woven bacon.
7. Line a baking sheet with kitchen foil and add plenty of salt to it.
8. Put the bacon on top of a cooling rack and put that on top of the baking sheet.
9. Bake for 60 minutes.
10. Let cool for 15 minutes before slicing and serve.

Cheese Crusted Chops

Prep time: 10 minutes | Cook time: 12 minutes | Serves 4 to 6

¼ teaspoon pepper

½ teaspoons salt

4 to 6 thick boneless pork chops

1 cup pork rind crumbs

¼ teaspoon chili powder

½ teaspoons onion powder

1 teaspoon smoked paprika

2 beaten eggs

3 tablespoons grated Parmesan cheese

Cooking spray

1. Set the temperature of the air fryer oven to 400ºF (205ºC). Press Start to begin preheating.
2. Rub the pepper and salt on both sides of pork chops.
3. In a food processor, pulse pork rinds into crumbs. Mix crumbs with chili powder, onion powder, and paprika in a bowl.
4. Beat eggs in another bowl.
5. Dip pork chops into eggs then into pork rind crumb mixture.
6. Spritz the air fryer oven with cooking spray and add pork chops to the perforated pan.
7. Air fry for 12 minutes.
8. Serve garnished with the Parmesan cheese.

Cheesy Beef Meatballs

Prep time: 5 minutes | Cook time: 18 minutes | Serves 6

1 pound (454 g) ground beef

½ cup grated Parmesan cheese

1 tablespoon minced garlic

½ cup Mozzarella cheese

1 teaspoon freshly ground pepper

1. Set the temperature of the air fryer oven to 400ºF (204ºC). Press Start to begin preheating.
2. In a bowl, mix all the ingredients together.
3. Roll the meat mixture into 5 generous meatballs.
4. Air fry inside the air fryer oven at 165ºF (74ºC) for about 18 minutes.
5. Serve immediately.

Chicken Fried Steak

Prep time: 15 minutes | Cook time: 10 minutes | Serves 4

½ cup flour

2 teaspoons salt, divided

Freshly ground black pepper, to taste

¼ teaspoon garlic powder

1 cup buttermilk

1 cup fine bread crumbs

4 (6-ounce / 170-g) tenderized top round steaks, ½-inch thick

Vegetable or canola oil

For the Gravy:

2 tablespoons butter or bacon drippings

¼ onion, minced

1 clove garlic, smashed

¼ teaspoon dried thyme

3 tablespoons flour

1 cup milk

Salt and freshly ground black pepper, to taste

Dashes of Worcestershire sauce

1. Set up a dredging station. Combine the flour, 1 teaspoon of salt, black pepper and garlic powder in a shallow

bowl. Pour the buttermilk into a second shallow bowl. Finally, put the bread crumbs and 1 teaspoon of salt in a third shallow bowl.

2. Dip the tenderized steaks into the flour, then the buttermilk, and then the bread crumb mixture, pressing the crumbs onto the steak. Put them on a baking sheet and spray both sides generously with vegetable or canola oil.
3. Set the temperature of the air fryer oven to 400ºF (204ºC). Press Start to begin preheating.
4. Transfer the steaks to the air fryer oven perforated pan, two at a time, and air fry for 10 minutes, flipping the steaks over halfway through the cooking time.
5. While the steaks are cooking, make the gravy. Melt the butter in a small saucepan over medium heat on the stovetop. Add the onion, garlic and thyme and cook for five minutes, until the onion is soft and just starting to brown. Stir in the flour and cook for another five minutes, stirring regularly, until the mixture starts to brown. Whisk in the milk and bring the mixture to a boil to thicken. Season to taste with salt, lots of freshly ground black pepper, and a few dashes of Worcestershire sauce.
6. Pour the gravy over the chicken fried steaks and serve.

Citrus Pork Loin Roast

Prep time: 10 minutes | Cook time: 45 minutes | Serves 8

1 tablespoon lime juice

1 tablespoon orange marmalade

1 teaspoon coarse brown mustard

1 teaspoon curry powder

1 teaspoon dried lemongrass

2 pound (907 g) boneless pork loin roast

Salt and ground black pepper, to taste

Cooking spray

1. Set the temperature of the air fryer oven to 360ºF (182ºC). Press Start to begin preheating.
2. Mix the lime juice, marmalade, mustard, curry powder, and lemongrass.
3. Rub mixture all over the surface of the pork loin. Season with salt and pepper.
4. Spray air fryer oven perforated pan with cooking spray and place pork roast diagonally in the perforated pan.
5. Air fry for approximately 45 minutes, until the internal temperature reaches at least 145ºF (63ºC).
6. Wrap roast in foil and let rest for 10 minutes before slicing.
7. Serve immediately.

Easy Beef Schnitzel

Prep time: 5 minutes | Cook time: 12 minutes | Serves 1

1 thin beef schnitzel

1 egg, beaten

½ cup friendly bread crumbs

2 tablespoons olive oil

Pepper and salt to taste

1. Set the temperature of the air fryer oven to 350ºF (177ºC). Press Start to begin preheating.
2. In a shallow dish, combine the bread crumbs, oil, pepper, and salt.
3. In a second shallow dish, place the beaten egg.
4. Dredge the schnitzel in the egg before rolling it in the bread crumbs.
5. Put the coated schnitzel in the air fryer oven perforated pan and air fry for 12 minutes. Flip the schnitzel halfway through.
6. Serve immediately.

Fast Lamb Satay

Prep time: 5 minutes | Cook time: 8 minutes | Serves 2

¼ teaspoon cumin

1 teaspoon ginger

½ teaspoons nutmeg

Salt and ground black pepper, to taste

2 boneless lamb steaks

Cooking spray

1. Combine the cumin, ginger, nutmeg, salt and pepper in a bowl.
2. Cube the lamb steaks and massage the spice mixture into each one.
3. Leave to marinate for 10 minutes, then transfer onto metal skewers.
4. Set the temperature of the air fryer oven to 400ºF (204ºC). Press Start to begin preheating.
5. Spritz the skewers with the cooking spray, then air fry them in the air fryer oven for 8 minutes.
6. Take care when removing them from the air fryer oven and serve.

Greek Lamb Pita Pockets

Prep time: 15 minutes | Cook time: 6 minutes | Serves 4

Dressing:

1 cup plain yogurt

1 tablespoon lemon juice

1 teaspoon dried dill weed, crushed

1 teaspoon ground oregano

½ teaspoon salt

Meatballs:

½ pound (227 g) ground lamb

1 tablespoon diced onion

1 teaspoon dried parsley

1 teaspoon dried dill weed, crushed

¼ teaspoon oregano

¼ teaspoon coriander

¼ teaspoon ground cumin

¼ teaspoon salt

4 pita halves

Suggested Toppings:

1 red onion, slivered

1 medium cucumber, deseeded, thinly sliced

Crumbled Feta cheese

Sliced black olives

Chopped fresh peppers

1. Set the temperature of the air fryer oven to 390ºF (199ºC). Press Start to begin preheating.
2. Stir the dressing ingredients together in a small bowl and refrigerate while preparing lamb.
3. Combine all meatball ingredients in a large bowl and stir to distribute seasonings.
4. Shape meat mixture into 12 small meatballs, rounded or slightly flattened if you prefer.
5. Transfer the meatballs in the preheated air fryer oven and air fry for 6 minutes, until well done. Remove and drain on paper towels.
6. To serve, pile meatballs and the choice of toppings in pita pockets and drizzle with dressing.

Greek Lamb Rack

Prep time: 5 minutes | Cook time: 10 minutes | Serves 4

¼ cup freshly squeezed lemon juice

1 teaspoon oregano

2 teaspoons minced fresh rosemary

1 teaspoon minced fresh thyme

2 tablespoons minced garlic

Salt and freshly ground black pepper, to taste

2 to 4 tablespoons olive oil

1 lamb rib rack (7 to 8 ribs)

1. Set the temperature of the air fryer oven to 360ºF (182ºC). Press Start to begin preheating.
2. In a small mixing bowl, combine the lemon juice, oregano, rosemary, thyme, garlic, salt, pepper, and olive oil and mix well.
3. Rub the mixture over the lamb, covering all the meat. Put the rack of lamb in the air fryer oven. Roast for 10 minutes. Flip the rack halfway through.
4. After 10 minutes, measure the internal temperature of the rack of lamb reaches at least 145ºF (63ºC).
5. Serve immediately.

Hearty Sweet and Sour Pork

Prep time: 20 minutes | Cook time: 14 minutes | Serves 2 to 4

1/3 cup all-purpose flour

⅓ cup cornstarch

2 teaspoons Chinese five-spice powder

1 teaspoon salt

Freshly ground black pepper, to taste

1 egg

2 tablespoons milk

¾ pound (340 g) boneless pork, cut into 1-inch cubes

Vegetable or canola oil

1½ cups large chunks of red and green peppers

½ cup ketchup

2 tablespoons rice wine vinegar or apple cider vinegar

2 tablespoons brown sugar

¼ cup orange juice

1 tablespoon soy sauce

1 clove garlic, minced

1 cup cubed pineapple

Chopped scallions, for garnish

1. Set up a dredging station with two bowls. Combine the flour, cornstarch, Chinese five-spice powder, salt and pepper in one large bowl. Whisk the egg and milk together in a second bowl. Dredge the pork cubes in the flour mixture first, then dip them into the egg and then back into the flour to coat on all sides. Spray the coated pork cubes with vegetable or canola oil.
2. Set the temperature of the air fryer oven to 400ºF (204ºC). Press Start to begin preheating.
3. Toss the pepper chunks with a little oil and air fry for 5 minutes, shaking the perforated pan halfway through the cooking time.
4. While the peppers are cooking, start making the sauce. Combine the ketchup, rice wine vinegar, brown sugar, orange juice, soy sauce, and garlic in a medium saucepan and bring the mixture to a boil on the stovetop. Reduce the heat and simmer for 5 minutes. When the peppers have finished air frying, add them to the saucepan along with the pineapple chunks. Simmer the peppers and pineapple in the sauce for an additional 2 minutes. Set aside and keep warm.
5. Add the dredged pork cubes to the air fryer oven perforated pan and air fry at 400ºF (204ºC) for 6

minutes, shaking the perforated pan to turn the cubes over for the last minute of the cooking process.

6. When ready to serve, toss the cooked pork with the pineapple, peppers and sauce. Serve garnished with chopped scallions.

Herbed Beef

Prep time: 5 minutes | Cook time: 22 minutes | Serves 6

1 teaspoon dried dill

1 teaspoon dried thyme

1 teaspoon garlic powder

2 pounds (907 g) beef steak

3 tablespoons butter

1. Set the temperature of the air fryer oven to 360ºF (182ºC). Press Start to begin preheating.
2. Combine the dill, thyme, and garlic powder together in a small bowl, and massage into the steak.
3. Air fry the steak in the air fryer oven for 20 minutes, then remove, shred, and return to the air fryer oven.
4. Add the butter and air fry the shredded steak for a further 2 minutes. Make sure the beef is coated in the butter before serving.

Italian Lamb Chops with Avocados Mayo

Prep time: 5 minutes | Cook time: 12 minutes | Serves 2

2 lamp chops

2 teaspoons Italian herbs

2 avocados

½ cup mayonnaise

1 tablespoon lemon juice

1. Season the lamb chops with the Italian herbs, then set aside for 5 minutes.
2. Set the temperature of the air fryer oven to 400ºF (204ºC) and place the rack inside.
3. Put the chops on the rack and air fry for 12 minutes.
4. In the meantime, halve the avocados and open to remove the pits. Spoon the flesh into a blender.
5. Add the mayonnaise and lemon juice and pulse until a smooth consistency is achieved.
6. Take care when removing the chops from the air fryer oven, then plate up and serve with the avocado mayo.

Kale and Beef Omelet

Prep time: 15 minutes | Cook time: 16 minutes | Serves 4

½ pound (227 g) leftover beef, coarsely chopped

2 garlic cloves, pressed

1 cup kale, torn into pieces and wilted

1 tomato, chopped

¼ teaspoon sugar

4 eggs, beaten

4 tablespoons heavy cream

½ teaspoon turmeric powder

Salt and ground black pepper, to taste

⅛ teaspoon ground allspice

Cooking spray

1. Set the temperature of the air fryer oven to 360ºF (182ºC). Press Start to begin preheating. Spritz four ramekins with cooking spray.
2. Put equal amounts of each of the ingredients into each ramekin and mix well.
3. Air fry for 16 minutes. Serve immediately.

Kielbasa Sausage with Pierogies

Prep time: 15 minutes | Cook time: 30 minutes | Serves 3 to 4

1 sweet onion, sliced

1 teaspoon olive oil

Salt and freshly ground black pepper, to taste

2 tablespoons butter, cut into small cubes

1 teaspoon sugar

1 pound (454 g) light Polish kielbasa sausage, cut into 2-inch chunks

1 (13-ounce / 369-g) package frozen mini pierogies

2 teaspoons vegetable or olive oil

Chopped scallions, for garnish

1. Set the temperature of the air fryer oven to 400ºF (204ºC). Press Start to begin preheating.
2. Toss the sliced onions with olive oil, salt and pepper and transfer them to the air fryer oven perforated pan. Dot the onions with pieces of butter and air fry for 2 minutes. Then sprinkle the sugar over the onions and stir. Pour any melted butter from the bottom of the air fryer oven drawer over the onions. Continue to air fry for another 13 minutes, stirring or shaking the perforated pan every few minutes to air fry the onions evenly.

3. Add the kielbasa chunks to the onions and toss. Air fry for another 5 minutes, shaking the perforated pan halfway through the cooking time. Transfer the kielbasa and onions to a bowl and cover with aluminum foil to keep warm.
4. Toss the frozen pierogies with the vegetable or olive oil and transfer them to the air fryer oven perforated pan. Air fry at 400ºF (204ºC) for 8 minutes, shaking the perforated pan twice during the cooking time.
5. When the pierogies have finished cooking, return the kielbasa and onions to the air fryer oven and gently toss with the pierogies. Air fry for 2 more minutes and then transfer everything to a serving platter. Garnish with the chopped scallions and serve hot with the spicy sour cream sauce below.

Lamb Burger

Prep time: 15 minutes | Cook time: 16 minutes | Serves 3 to 4

2 teaspoons olive oil

⅓ onion, finely chopped

1 clove garlic, minced

1 pound (454 g) ground lamb

2 tablespoons fresh parsley, finely chopped

1½ teaspoons fresh oregano, finely chopped

½ cup black olives, finely chopped

⅓ cup crumbled feta cheese

½ teaspoon salt

freshly ground black pepper

4 thick pita breads

toppings and condiments

1. Preheat a medium skillet over medium-high heat on the stovetop. Add the olive oil and cook the onion until tender, but not browned – about 4 to 5 minutes. Add the garlic and cook for another minute. Transfer the onion and garlic to a mixing bowl and add the ground lamb, parsley, oregano, olives, feta cheese, salt and pepper. Gently mix the ingredients together.

2. Divide the mixture into 3 or 4 equal portions and then form the hamburgers, being careful not to over-handle the meat. One good way to do this is to throw the meat back and forth between the hands like a baseball, packing the meat each time you catch it. Flatten the balls into patties, making an indentation in the center of each patty. Flatten the sides of the patties.
3. Set the temperature of the air fryer oven to 370ºF (188ºC). Press Start to begin preheating.
4. If you don't have room for all four burgers, air fry two or three burgers at a time for 8 minutes. Flip the burgers over and air fry for another 8 minutes. If you cooked the burgers in batches, return the first batch of burgers to the air fryer oven for the last two minutes of cooking to re-heat. This should give you a medium-well burger. If you'd prefer a medium-rare burger, shorten the cooking time to about 13 minutes. Remove the burgers to a resting plate and let the burgers rest for a few minutes before dressing and serving.
5. While the burgers are resting, toast the pita breads in the air fryer oven for 2 minutes. Tuck the burgers into the toasted pita breads, or wrap the pitas around the burgers and serve with a tzatziki sauce or some mayonnaise.

Lamb Meatballs

Prep time: 20 minutes | Cook time: 8 minutes | Serves 4

Meatballs:

½ small onion, finely diced

1 clove garlic, minced

1 pound (454 g) ground lamb

2 tablespoons fresh parsley, finely chopped (plus more for garnish)

2 teaspoons fresh oregano, finely chopped

2 tablespoons milk

1 egg yolk

Salt and freshly ground black pepper, to taste

½ cup crumbled feta cheese, for garnish

Tomato Sauce:

2 tablespoons butter

1 clove garlic, smashed

Pinch crushed red pepper flakes

¼ teaspoon ground cinnamon

1 (28-ounce / 794-g) can crushed tomatoes

Salt, to taste

Olive oil, for greasing

1. Combine all ingredients for the meatballs in a large bowl and mix just until everything is combined. Shape the mixture into 1½-inch balls or shape the meat between two spoons to make quenelles.
2. Set the temperature of the air fryer oven to 400ºF (204ºC). Press Start to begin preheating.
3. While the air fryer oven is preheating, start the quick tomato sauce. Put the butter, garlic and red pepper flakes in a sauté pan and heat over medium heat on the stovetop. Let the garlic sizzle a little, but before the butter browns, add the cinnamon and tomatoes. Bring to a simmer and simmer for 15 minutes. Season with salt.
4. Grease the bottom of the air fryer oven perforated pan with olive oil and transfer the meatballs to the air fryer oven perforated pan in one layer, air frying in batches if necessary.
5. Air fry for 8 minutes, giving the perforated pan a shake once during the cooking process to turn the meatballs over.
6. To serve, spoon a pool of the tomato sauce onto plates and add the meatballs. Sprinkle the feta cheese on top and garnish with more fresh parsley. Serve immediately.

Lollipop Lamb Chops

Prep time: 15 minutes | Cook time: 7 minutes | Serves 4

½ small clove garlic

¼ cup packed fresh parsley

¾ cup packed fresh mint

½ teaspoon lemon juice

¼ cup grated Parmesan cheese

⅓ cup shelled pistachios

¼ teaspoon salt

½ cup olive oil

8 lamb chops (1 rack)

2 tablespoons vegetable oil

Salt and freshly ground black pepper, to taste

1 tablespoon dried rosemary, chopped

1 tablespoon dried thyme

1. Make the pesto by combining the garlic, parsley and mint in a food processor and process until finely chopped. Add the lemon juice, Parmesan cheese, pistachios and salt. Process until all the ingredients have turned into a paste. With the processor running, slowly pour the olive oil in. Scrape the sides of the processor with a spatula and process for another 30 seconds.
2. Set the temperature of the air fryer oven to 400ºF (204ºC). Press Start to begin preheating.
3. Rub both sides of the lamb chops with vegetable oil and season with salt, pepper, rosemary and thyme, pressing the herbs into the meat gently with the fingers. Transfer the lamb chops to the air fryer oven perforated pan.
4. Air fry the lamb chops for 5 minutes. Flip the chops over and air fry for an additional 2 minutes.
5. Serve the lamb chops with mint pesto drizzled on top.

Marinated Pork Tenderloin

Prep time: 10 minutes | Cook time: 30 minutes | Serves 4 to 6

¼ cup olive oil

¼ cup soy sauce

¼ cup freshly squeezed lemon juice

1 garlic clove, minced

1 tablespoon Dijon mustard

1 teaspoon salt

½ teaspoon freshly ground black pepper

2 pounds (907 g) pork tenderloin

1. In a large mixing bowl, make the marinade: Mix the olive oil, soy sauce, lemon juice, minced garlic, Dijon mustard, salt, and pepper. Reserve ¼ cup of the marinade.
2. Put the tenderloin in a large bowl and pour the remaining marinade over the meat. Cover and marinate in the refrigerator for about 1 hour.
3. Set the temperature of the air fryer oven to 400ºF (204ºC). Press Start to begin preheating.
4. Put the marinated pork tenderloin into the air fryer oven perforated pan. Roast for 10 minutes. Flip the pork and baste it with half of the reserved marinade. Roast for 10 minutes more.
5. Flip the pork, then baste with the remaining marinade. Roast for another 10 minutes, for a total cooking time of 30 minutes.
6. Serve immediately.

Mexican Pork Chops

Prep time: 5 minutes | Cook time: 15 minutes | Serves 2

¼ teaspoon dried oregano

1½ teaspoons taco seasoning mix

2 (4-ounce / 113-g) boneless pork chops

2 tablespoons unsalted butter, divided

1. Set the temperature of the air fryer oven to 400ºF (204ºC). Press Start to begin preheating.
2. Combine the dried oregano and taco seasoning in a small bowl and rub the mixture into the pork chops. Brush the chops with 1 tablespoon butter.
3. In the air fryer oven, air fry the chops for 15 minutes, turning them over halfway through to air fry on the other side.
4. When the chops are a brown color, check the internal temperature has reached 145ºF (63ºC) and remove from the air fryer oven. Serve with a garnish of remaining butter.

Miso Marinated Steak

Prep time: 5 minutes | Cook time: 12 minutes | Serves 4

¾ pound (340 g) flank steak

1½ tablespoons sake

1 tablespoon brown miso paste

1 teaspoon honey

2 cloves garlic, pressed

1 tablespoon olive oil

1. Put all the ingredients in a Ziploc bag. Shake to cover the steak well with the seasonings and refrigerate for at least 1 hour.
2. Set the temperature of the air fryer oven to 400ºF (204ºC). Press Start to begin preheating. Coat all sides of the steak with cooking spray. Put the steak in the baking pan.
3. Air fry for 12 minutes, turning the steak twice during the cooking time, then serve immediately.

Mongolian Flank Steak

Prep time: 20 minutes | Cook time: 15 minutes | Serves 4

1½ pounds (680 g) flank steak, thinly sliced on the bias into ¼-inch strips

Marinade:

2 tablespoons soy sauce

1 clove garlic, smashed

Pinch crushed red pepper flakes

Sauce:

1 tablespoon vegetable oil

2 cloves garlic, minced

1 tablespoon finely grated fresh ginger

3 dried red chili peppers

¾ cup soy sauce

¾ cup chicken stock

5 to 6 tablespoons brown sugar

½ cup cornstarch, divided

1 bunch scallions, sliced into 2-inch pieces

1. Marinate the beef in the soy sauce, garlic and red pepper flakes for one hour.
2. In the meantime, make the sauce. Preheat a small saucepan over medium heat on the stovetop. Add the oil,

garlic, ginger and dried chili peppers and sauté for just a minute or two. Add the soy sauce, chicken stock and brown sugar and continue to simmer for a few minutes. Dissolve 3 tablespoons of cornstarch in 3 tablespoons of water and stir this into the saucepan. Stir the sauce over medium heat until it thickens. Set this aside.

3. Set the temperature of the air fryer oven to 400ºF (204ºC). Press Start to begin preheating.
4. Remove the beef from the marinade and transfer it to a zipper sealable plastic bag with the remaining cornstarch. Shake it around to completely coat the beef and transfer the coated strips of beef to a baking sheet or plate, shaking off any excess cornstarch. Spray the strips with vegetable oil on all sides and transfer them to the air fryer oven perforated pan.
5. Air fry for 15 minutes, shaking the perforated pan to toss and rotate the beef strips throughout the cooking process. Add the scallions for the last 4 minutes of the cooking. Transfer the hot beef strips and scallions to a bowl and toss with the sauce, coating all the beef strips with the sauce. Serve warm.

Mozzarella Beef Brisket

Prep time: 5 minutes | Cook time: 25 minutes | Serves 6

12 ounces (340 g) beef brisket

2 teaspoons Italian herbs

2 teaspoons butter

1 onion, sliced

7 ounces (198 g) Mozzarella cheese, sliced

1. Set the temperature of the air fryer oven to 365ºF (185ºC). Press Start to begin preheating.
2. Cut up the brisket into four equal slices and season with the Italian herbs.
3. Allow the butter to melt in the air fryer oven. Put the slices of beef inside along with the onion. Air fry for 25 minutes. Flip the brisket halfway through. Put a piece of Mozzarella on top of each piece of brisket in the last 5 minutes.
4. Serve immediately.

Mushroom and Beef Meatloaf

Prep time: 10 minutes | Cook time: 25 minutes | Serves 4

1 pound (454 g) ground beef

1 egg, beaten

1 mushrooms, sliced

1 tablespoon thyme

1 small onion, chopped

3 tablespoons bread crumbs

Ground black pepper, to taste

1. Set the temperature of the air fryer oven to 400ºF (204ºC). Press Start to begin preheating.
2. Put all the ingredients into a large bowl and combine entirely.
3. Transfer the meatloaf mixture into the loaf pan and move it to the air fryer oven.
4. Bake for 25 minutes. Slice up before serving.

Orange Pork Tenderloin

Prep time: 15 minutes | Cook time: 23 minutes | Serves 3 to 4

2 tablespoons brown sugar

2 teaspoons cornstarch

2 teaspoons Dijon mustard

½ cup orange juice

½ teaspoon soy sauce

2 teaspoons grated fresh ginger

¼ cup white wine

Zest of 1 orange

1 pound (454 g) pork tenderloin

Salt and freshly ground black pepper, to taste

Oranges, halved, for garnish

Fresh parsley, for garnish

1. Combine the brown sugar, cornstarch, Dijon mustard, orange juice, soy sauce, ginger, white wine and orange zest in a small saucepan and bring the mixture to a boil on the stovetop. Lower the heat and simmer while you air fry the pork tenderloin or until the sauce has thickened.
2. Set the temperature of the air fryer oven to 370ºF (188ºC). Press Start to begin preheating.

3. Season all sides of the pork tenderloin with salt and freshly ground black pepper. Transfer the tenderloin to the air fryer oven perforated pan.
4. Air fry for 20 to 23 minutes, or until the internal temperature reaches 145ºF (63ºC). Flip the tenderloin over halfway through the cooking process and baste with the sauce.
5. Transfer the tenderloin to a cutting board and let it rest for 5 minutes. Slice the pork at a slight angle and serve immediately with orange halves and fresh parsley.
6. Serve immediately.

Peppercorn Crusted Beef Tenderloin

Prep time: 5 minutes | Cook time: 25 minutes | Serves 6

2 pounds (907 g) beef tenderloin

2 teaspoons roasted garlic, minced

2 tablespoons salted butter, melted

3 tablespoons ground 4-peppercorn blender

1. Set the temperature of the air fryer oven to 400ºF (204ºC). Press Start to begin preheating.
2. Remove any surplus fat from the beef tenderloin.
3. Combine the roasted garlic and melted butter to apply to the tenderloin with a brush.
4. On a plate, spread out the peppercorns and roll the tenderloin in them, making sure they are covering and clinging to the meat.
5. Air fry the tenderloin in the air fryer oven for 25 minutes, turning halfway through cooking.
6. Let the tenderloin rest for ten minutes before slicing and serving.

Pepperoni and Bell Pepper Pockets

Prep time: 5 minutes | Cook time: 8 minutes | Serves 4

4 bread slices, 1-inch thick

Olive oil, for misting

24 slices pepperoni

1 ounce (28 g) roasted red peppers, drained and patted dry

1 ounce (28 g) Pepper Jack cheese, cut into 4 slices

1. Set the temperature of the air fryer oven to 360ºF (182ºC). Press Start to begin preheating.
2. Spray both sides of bread slices with olive oil.
3. Stand slices upright and cut a deep slit in the top to create a pocket (almost to the bottom crust, but not all the way through).
4. Stuff each bread pocket with 6 slices of pepperoni, a large strip of roasted red pepper, and a slice of cheese.
5. Put bread pockets in air fryer oven perforated pan, standing up. Air fry for 8 minutes, until filling is heated through and bread is lightly browned.
6. Serve hot.

Pork and Pinto Bean Gorditas

Prep time: 20 minutes | Cook time: 21 minutes | Serves 4

1 pound (454 g) lean ground pork

2 tablespoons chili powder

2 tablespoons ground cumin

1 teaspoon dried oregano

2 teaspoons paprika

1 teaspoon garlic powder

½ cup water

1 (15-ounce / 425-g) can pinto beans, drained and rinsed

½ cup taco sauce

Salt and freshly ground black pepper, to taste

2 cups grated Cheddar cheese

5 (12-inch) flour tortillas

4 (8-inch) crispy corn tortilla shells

4 cups shredded lettuce

1 tomato, diced

⅓ cup sliced black olives

Sour cream, for serving

Tomato salsa, for serving

Cooking spray

1. Set the temperature of the air fryer oven to 400ºF (204ºC). Press Start to begin preheating. Spritz the perforated pan with cooking spray.
2. Put the ground pork in the perforated pan and air fry at 400ºF (204ºC) for 10 minutes, stirring a few times to gently break up the meat. Combine the chili powder, cumin, oregano, paprika, garlic powder and water in a small bowl. Stir the spice mixture into the browned pork. Stir in the beans and taco sauce and air fry for an additional minute. Transfer the pork mixture to a bowl. Season with salt and freshly ground black pepper.
3. Sprinkle ½ cup of the grated cheese in the center of the flour tortillas, leaving a 2-inch border around the edge free of cheese and filling. Divide the pork mixture among the four tortillas, placing it on top of the cheese. Put a crunchy corn tortilla on top of the pork and top with shredded lettuce, diced tomatoes, and black olives. Cut the remaining flour tortilla into 4 quarters. These quarters of tortilla will serve as the bottom of the gordita. Put one quarter tortilla on top of each gordita and fold the edges of the bottom flour tortilla up over the sides, enclosing the filling. While holding the seams down, brush the bottom of the gordita with olive oil and place the seam side down on the countertop while you finish the remaining three gorditas.

4. Set the temperature of the air fryer oven to 380ºF (193ºC). Press Start to begin preheating.
5. Air fry one gordita at a time. Transfer the gordita carefully to the air fryer oven perforated pan, seam side down. Brush or spray the top tortilla with oil and air fry for 5 minutes. Carefully turn the gordita over and air fry for an additional 4 to 5 minutes until both sides are browned. When finished air frying all four gorditas, layer them back into the air fryer oven for an additional minute to make sure they are all warm before serving with sour cream and salsa.

Pork Chop Stir Fry

Prep time: 10 minutes | Cook time: 20 minutes | Serves 4

1 tablespoon olive oil

¼ teaspoon ground black pepper

½ teaspoon salt

1 egg white

4 (4-ounce / 113-g) pork chops

¾ cup almond flour

2 sliced jalapeño peppers

2 sliced scallions

2 tablespoons olive oil

¼ teaspoon ground white pepper

1 teaspoon sea salt

1. Coat the air fryer oven perforated pan with olive oil.
2. Whisk black pepper, salt, and egg white together until foamy.
3. Cut pork chops into pieces, leaving just a bit on bones. Pat dry.
4. Add pieces of pork to egg white mixture, coating well. Let sit for marinade 20 minutes.
5. Set the temperature of the air fryer oven to 360ºF (182ºC). Press Start to begin preheating.

6. Put marinated chops into a large bowl and add almond flour. Dredge and shake off excess and place into air fryer oven.
7. Air fry the chops in the preheated air fryer oven for 12 minutes.
8. Turn up the heat to 400ºF (205ºC) and air fry for another 6 minutes until pork chops are nice and crisp.
9. Meanwhile, remove the jalapeño seeds and chop up. Chop scallions and mix with jalapeño pieces.
10. Heat a skillet with olive oil. Stir-fry the white pepper, salt, scallions, and jalapeños 60 seconds. Then add fried pork pieces to skills and toss with scallion mixture. Stir-fry 1 to 2 minutes until well coated and hot.
11. Serve immediately.

Pork Chops with Rinds

Prep time: 5 minutes | Cook time: 15 minutes | Serves 4

1 teaspoon chili powder

½ teaspoon garlic powder

1½ ounces (43 g) pork rinds, finely ground

4 (4-ounce / 113-g) pork chops

1 tablespoon coconut oil, melted

1. Set the temperature of the air fryer oven to 400ºF (204ºC). Press Start to begin preheating.
2. Combine the chili powder, garlic powder, and ground pork rinds.
3. Coat the pork chops with the coconut oil, followed by the pork rind mixture, taking care to cover them completely. Then place the chops in the perforated pan of the air fryer oven.
4. Air fry the chops for 15 minutes or until the internal temperature of the chops reaches at least 145ºF (63ºC), turning halfway through.
5. Serve immediately.

Pork Medallions with Radicchio and Endive Salad

Prep time: 25 minutes | Cook time: 7 minutes | Serves 4

1 (8-ounce / 227-g) pork tenderloin

Salt and freshly ground black pepper, to taste

¼ cup flour

2 eggs, lightly beaten

¾ cup cracker meal

1 teaspoon paprika

1 teaspoon dry mustard

1 teaspoon garlic powder

1 teaspoon dried thyme

1 teaspoon salt

vegetable or canola oil, in spray bottle

Vinaigrette:

¼ cup white balsamic vinegar

2 tablespoons agave syrup (or honey or maple syrup)

1 tablespoon Dijon mustard

juice of ½ lemon

2 tablespoons chopped chervil or flat-leaf parsley

salt and freshly ground black pepper

½ cup extra-virgin olive oil

Radicchio and Endive Salad:

1 heart romaine lettuce, torn into large pieces

½ head radicchio, coarsely chopped

2 heads endive, sliced

½ cup cherry tomatoes, halved

3 ounces (85 g) fresh Mozzarella, diced

Salt and freshly ground black pepper, to taste

1. Slice the pork tenderloin into 1-inch slices. Using a meat pounder, pound the pork slices into thin ½-inch medallions. Generously season the pork with salt and freshly ground black pepper on both sides.
2. Set up a dredging station using three shallow dishes. Put the flour in one dish and the beaten eggs in a second dish. Combine the cracker meal, paprika, dry mustard, garlic powder, thyme and salt in a third dish.
3. Set the temperature of the air fryer oven to 400ºF (204ºC). Press Start to begin preheating.
4. Dredge the pork medallions in flour first and then into the beaten egg. Let the excess egg drip off and coat both sides of the medallions with the cracker meal crumb mixture. Spray both sides of the coated medallions with vegetable or canola oil.
5. Air fry the medallions in two batches at 400ºF (204ºC) for 5 minutes. Once you have air-fried all the medallions, flip them all over and return the first batch of medallions

back into the air fryer oven on top of the second batch. Air fry at 400ºF (204ºC) for an additional 2 minutes.

6. While the medallions are cooking, make the salad and dressing. Whisk the white balsamic vinegar, agave syrup, Dijon mustard, lemon juice, chervil, salt and pepper together in a small bowl. Whisk in the olive oil slowly until combined and thickened.
7. Combine the romaine lettuce, radicchio, endive, cherry tomatoes, and Mozzarella cheese in a large salad bowl. Drizzle the dressing over the vegetables and toss to combine. Season with salt and freshly ground black pepper.
8. Serve the pork medallions warm on or beside the salad.

Pork with Aloha Salsa

Prep time: 20 minutes | Cook time: 8 minutes | Serves 4

2 eggs

2 tablespoons milk

¼ cup flour

¼ cup panko bread crumbs

4 teaspoons sesame seeds

1 pound (454 g) boneless, thin pork cutlets (⅜- to ½-inch thick)

Lemon pepper and salt, to taste

¼ cup cornstarch

Cooking spray

Aloha Salsa:

1 cup fresh pineapple, chopped in small pieces

¼ cup red onion, finely chopped

¼ cup green or red bell pepper, chopped

½ teaspoon ground cinnamon

1 teaspoon low-sodium soy sauce

⅛ teaspoon crushed red pepper

⅛ teaspoon ground black pepper

1. In a medium bowl, stir together all ingredients for salsa. Cover and refrigerate while cooking the pork.

2. Set the temperature of the air fryer oven to 390ºF (199ºC). Press Start to begin preheating.
3. Beat the eggs and milk in a shallow dish.
4. In another shallow dish, mix the flour, panko, and sesame seeds.
5. Sprinkle pork cutlets with lemon pepper and salt.
6. Dip pork cutlets in cornstarch, egg mixture, and then panko coating. Spray both sides with cooking spray.
7. Air fry the cutlets for 3 minutes. Turn cutlets over, spraying both sides, and continue air frying for 5 minutes or until well done.
8. Serve fried cutlets with salsa on the side.

Potato and Prosciutto Salad

Prep time: 10 minutes | Cook time: 7 minutes | Serves 8

Salad:

4 pounds (1.8 kg) potatoes, boiled and cubed

15 slices prosciutto, diced

2 cups shredded Cheddar cheese

Dressing:

15 ounces (425 g) sour cream

2 tablespoons mayonnaise

1 teaspoon salt

1 teaspoon black pepper

1 teaspoon dried basil

1. Set the temperature of the air fryer oven to 350ºF (177ºC). Press Start to begin preheating.
2. Put the potatoes, prosciutto, and Cheddar in a baking dish. Put it in the air fryer oven and air fry for 7 minutes.
3. In a separate bowl, mix the sour cream, mayonnaise, salt, pepper, and basil using a whisk.
4. Coat the salad with the dressing and serve.

Provolone Stuffed Beef and Pork Meatballs

Prep time: 15 minutes | Cook time: 12 minutes | Serves 4 to 6

1 tablespoon olive oil

1 small onion, finely chopped

1 to 2 cloves garlic, minced

¾ pound (340 g) ground beef

¾ pound (340 g) ground pork

¾ cup bread crumbs

¼ cup grated Parmesan cheese

¼ cup finely chopped fresh parsley

½ teaspoon dried oregano

1½ teaspoons salt

Freshly ground black pepper, to taste

2 eggs, lightly beaten

5 ounces (142 g) sharp or aged provolone cheese, cut into 1-inch cubes

1. Preheat a skillet over medium-high heat. Add the oil and cook the onion and garlic until tender, but not browned.
2. Transfer the onion and garlic to a large bowl and add the beef, pork, bread crumbs, Parmesan cheese, parsley, oregano, salt, pepper and eggs. Mix well until all the ingredients are combined. Divide the mixture into 12 evenly sized balls. Make one meatball at a time, by

pressing a hole in the meatball mixture with the finger and pushing a piece of provolone cheese into the hole. Mold the meat back into a ball, enclosing the cheese.

3. Set the temperature of the air fryer oven to 380ºF (193ºC). Press Start to begin preheating.
4. Working in two batches, transfer six of the meatballs to the air fryer oven perforated pan and air fry for 12 minutes, shaking the perforated pan and turning the meatballs twice during the cooking process. Repeat with the remaining 6 meatballs. Serve warm.

Ritzy Skirt Steak Fajitas

Prep time: 15 minutes | Cook time: 30 minutes | Serves 4

2 tablespoons olive oil

¼ cup lime juice

1 clove garlic, minced

½ teaspoon ground cumin

½ teaspoon hot sauce

½ teaspoon salt

2 tablespoons chopped fresh cilantro

1 pound (454 g) skirt steak

1 onion, sliced

1 teaspoon chili powder

1 red pepper, sliced

1 green pepper, sliced

Salt and freshly ground black pepper, to taste

8 flour tortillas

Toppings:

Shredded lettuce

Crumbled Queso Fresco (or grated Cheddar cheese)

Sliced black olives

Diced tomatoes

Sour cream

Guacamole

1. Combine the olive oil, lime juice, garlic, cumin, hot sauce, salt and cilantro in a shallow dish. Add the skirt steak and turn it over several times to coat all sides. Pierce the steak with a needle-style meat tenderizer or paring knife. Marinate the steak in the refrigerator for at least 3 hours, or overnight. When you are ready to cook, remove the steak from the refrigerator and let it sit at room temperature for 30 minutes.
2. Set the temperature of the air fryer oven to 400ºF (204ºC). Press Start to begin preheating.
3. Toss the onion slices with the chili powder and a little olive oil and transfer them to the air fryer oven perforated pan. Air fry for 5 minutes. Add the red and green peppers to the air fryer oven perforated pan with the onions, season with salt and pepper and air fry for 8 more minutes, until the onions and peppers are soft. Transfer the vegetables to a dish and cover with aluminum foil to keep warm.
4. Put the skirt steak in the air fryer oven perforated pan and pour the marinade over the top. Air fry at 400ºF (204ºC) for 12 minutes. Flip the steak over and air fry for an additional 5 minutes. Transfer the cooked steak to a cutting board and let the steak rest for a few

minutes. If the peppers and onions need to be heated, return them to the air fryer oven for just 1 to 2 minutes.

5. Thinly slice the steak at an angle, cutting against the grain of the steak. Serve the steak with the onions and peppers, the warm tortillas and the fajita toppings on the side.
6. Serve immediately.

Rosemary Ribeye Steaks

Prep time: 10 minutes | Cook time: 15 minutes | Serves 2

¼ cup butter

1 clove garlic, minced

Salt and ground black pepper, to taste

1½ tablespoons balsamic vinegar

¼ cup rosemary, chopped

2 ribeye steaks

1. Melt the butter in a skillet over medium heat. Add the garlic and fry until fragrant.
2. Remove the skillet from the heat and add the salt, pepper, and vinegar. Allow it to cool.
3. Add the rosemary, then pour the mixture into a Ziploc bag.
4. Put the ribeye steaks in the bag and shake well, coating the meat well. Refrigerate for an hour, then allow to sit for a further twenty minutes.
5. Set the temperature of the air fryer oven to 400ºF (204ºC) and set the rack inside. Air fry the ribeyes for 15 minutes.
6. Take care when removing the steaks from the air fryer oven and plate up.
7. Serve immediately.

Simple Pulled Pork

Prep time: 5 minutes | Cook time: 24 minutes | Serves 1

2 tablespoons barbecue dry rub

1 pound (454 g) pork tenderloin

⅓ cup heavy cream

1 teaspoon butter

1. Set the temperature of the air fryer oven to 370ºF (188ºC). Press Start to begin preheating.
2. Massage the dry rub into the tenderloin, coating it well.
3. Air fry the tenderloin in the air fryer oven for 20 minutes. When air fried, shred with two forks.
4. Add the heavy cream and butter into the air fryer oven along with the shredded pork and stir well. Air fry for a further 4 minutes.
5. Allow to cool, then serve.

Smoked Beef

Prep time: 10 minutes | Cook time: 45 minutes | Serves 8

2 pounds (907 g) roast beef, at room temperature

2 tablespoons extra-virgin olive oil

1 teaspoon sea salt flakes

1 teaspoon ground black pepper

1 teaspoon smoked paprika

Few dashes of liquid smoke

2 jalapeño peppers, thinly sliced

1. Set the temperature of the air fryer oven to 330ºF (166ºC). Press Start to begin preheating.
2. With kitchen towels, pat the beef dry.
3. Massage the extra-virgin olive oil, salt, black pepper, and paprika into the meat. Cover with liquid smoke.
4. Put the beef in the air fryer oven and roast for 30 minutes. Flip the roast over and allow to roast for another 15 minutes.
5. When cooked through, serve topped with sliced jalapeños.

Spaghetti Squash Lasagna

Prep time: 5 minutes | Cook time: 1 hour 15 minutes | Serves 6

2 large spaghetti squash, cooked (about 2¾ pounds / 1.2 kg)

4 pounds (1.8 kg) ground beef

1 (2½-pound / 1.1-kg) large jar Marinara sauce

25 slices Mozzarella cheese

30 ounces whole-milk ricotta cheese

1. Set the temperature of the air fryer oven to 375ºF (191ºC). Press Start to begin preheating.
2. Slice the spaghetti squash and place it face down inside a baking dish. Fill with water until covered.
3. Bake in the preheated air fryer oven for 45 minutes until skin is soft.
4. Sear the ground beef in a skillet over medium-high heat for 5 minutes or until browned, then add the marinara sauce and heat until warm. Set aside.
5. Scrape the flesh off the cooked squash to resemble strands of spaghetti.
6. Layer the lasagna in a large greased pan in alternating layers of spaghetti squash, beef sauce, Mozzarella, ricotta. Repeat until all the ingredients have been used.
7. Bake for 30 minutes and serve.

Spinach and Beef Braciole

Prep time: 25 minutes | Cook time: 1 hour 32 minutes | Serves 4

½ onion, finely chopped

1 teaspoon olive oil

⅓ cup red wine

2 cups crushed tomatoes

1 teaspoon Italian seasoning

½ teaspoon garlic powder

¼ teaspoon crushed red pepper flakes

2 tablespoons chopped fresh parsley

2 top round steaks (about 1½ pounds / 680 g)

salt and freshly ground black pepper

2 cups fresh spinach, chopped

1 clove minced garlic

½ cup roasted red peppers, julienned

½ cup grated pecorino cheese

¼ cup pine nuts, toasted and roughly chopped

2 tablespoons olive oil

1. Set the temperature of the air fryer oven to 400ºF (204ºC). Press Start to begin preheating.
2. Toss the onions and olive oil together in a baking pan. Air fry at 400ºF (204ºC) for 5 minutes, stirring a couple times during the cooking process. Add the red wine, crushed tomatoes, Italian seasoning, garlic powder, red pepper flakes and parsley and stir. Cover the pan tightly with aluminum foil, lower the air fryer oven temperature to 350ºF (177ºC) and continue to air fry for 15 minutes.
3. While the sauce is simmering, prepare the beef. Using a meat mallet, pound the beef until it is ¼-inch thick. Season both sides of the beef with salt and pepper. Combine the spinach, garlic, red peppers, pecorino cheese, pine nuts and olive oil in a medium bowl. Season with salt and freshly ground black pepper. Disperse the mixture over the steaks. Starting at one of the short ends, roll the beef around the filling, tucking in the sides as you roll to ensure the filling is completely enclosed. Secure the beef rolls with toothpicks.
4. Remove the baking pan with the sauce from the air fryer oven and set it aside. Set the temperature of the air fryer oven to 400ºF (204ºC). Press Start to begin preheating.

5. Brush or spray the beef rolls with a little olive oil and air fry at 400ºF (204ºC) for 12 minutes, rotating the beef during the cooking process for even browning. When the beef is browned, submerge the rolls into the sauce in the baking pan, cover the pan with foil and return it to the air fryer oven. Reduce the temperature of the air fryer oven to 250ºF (121ºC) and air fry for 60 minutes.
6. Remove the beef rolls from the sauce. Cut each roll into slices and serve, ladling some sauce overtop.

Sumptuous Pizza Tortilla Rolls

Prep time: 10 minutes | Cook time: 6 minutes | Serves 4

1 teaspoon butter

½ medium onion, slivered

½ red or green bell pepper, julienned

4 ounces (113 g) fresh white mushrooms, chopped

½ cup pizza sauce

8 flour tortillas

8 thin slices deli ham

24 pepperoni slices

1 cup shredded Mozzarella cheese

Cooking spray

1. Set the temperature of the air fryer oven to 390ºF (199ºC). Press Start to begin preheating.
2. Put butter, onions, bell pepper, and mushrooms in a baking pan. Bake in the preheated air fryer oven for 3 minutes. Stir and cook 3 to 4 minutes longer until just crisp and tender. Remove pan and set aside.
3. To assemble rolls, spread about 2 teaspoons of pizza sauce on one half of each tortilla. Top with a slice of ham and 3 slices of pepperoni. Divide sautéed vegetables among tortillas and top with cheese.

4. Roll up tortillas, secure with toothpicks if needed, and spray with oil.
5. Put 4 rolls in air fryer oven perforated pan and air fry for 4 minutes. Turn and air fry 4 minutes, until heated through and lightly browned.
6. Repeat step 4 to air fry remaining pizza rolls.
7. Serve immediately.

Sun-dried Tomato Crusted Chops

Prep time: 15 minutes | Cook time: 10 minutes | Serves 4

½ cup oil-packed sun-dried tomatoes

½ cup toasted almonds

¼ cup grated Parmesan cheese

½ cup olive oil, plus more for brushing the air fryer basket

2 tablespoons water

½ teaspoon salt

Freshly ground black pepper, to taste

4 center-cut boneless pork chops (about 1¼ pounds / 567 g)

1. Put the sun-dried tomatoes into a food processor and pulse them until they are coarsely chopped. Add the almonds, Parmesan cheese, olive oil, water, salt and pepper. Process into a smooth paste. Spread most of the paste (leave a little in reserve) onto both sides of the pork chops and then pierce the meat several times with a needle-style meat tenderizer or a fork. Let the pork chops sit and marinate for at least 1 hour (refrigerate if marinating for longer than 1 hour).
2. Set the temperature of the air fryer oven to 370ºF (188ºC). Press Start to begin preheating.
3. Brush more olive oil on the bottom of the air fryer oven perforated pan. Transfer the pork chops into the air

fryer oven perforated pan, spooning a little more of the sun-dried tomato paste onto the pork chops if there are any gaps where the paste may have been rubbed off. Air fry the pork chops for 10 minutes, turning the chops over halfway through.

4. When the pork chops have finished cooking, transfer them to a serving plate and serve.

Super Bacon with Meat

Prep time: 5 minutes | Cook time: 1 hour | Serves 4

30 slices thick-cut bacon

4 ounces (113 g) Cheddar cheese, shredded

12 ounces (340 g) steak

10 ounces (283 g) pork sausage

Salt and ground black pepper, to taste

1. Set the temperature of the air fryer oven to 400ºF (204ºC). Press Start to begin preheating.
2. Lay out 30 slices of bacon in a woven pattern in the perforated pan in the air fryer oven and bake for 20 minutes until crisp.
3. Combine the steak and sausage to form a meaty mixture.
4. Lay out the meat in a rectangle of similar size to the bacon strips. Season with salt and pepper. Put the cheese in the center.
5. Roll the meat into a tight roll and refrigerate.
6. Set the temperature of the air fryer oven to 400ºF (204ºC). Press Start to begin preheating.
7. Make a 7×7 bacon weave and roll the bacon weave over the meat, diagonally.
8. Bake for 60 minutes or until the internal temperature reaches at least 165ºF (74ºC).
9. Let rest for 5 minutes before serving.

Swedish Beef Meatballs

Prep time: 10 minutes | Cook time: 12 minutes | Serves 8

1 pound (454 g) ground beef

1 egg, beaten

2 carrots, shredded

2 bread slices, crumbled

1 small onion, minced

½ teaspoons garlic salt

Pepper and salt, to taste

1 cup tomato sauce

2 cups pasta sauce

1. Set the temperature of the air fryer oven to 400ºF (204ºC). Press Start to begin preheating.
2. In a bowl, combine the ground beef, egg, carrots, crumbled bread, onion, garlic salt, pepper and salt.
3. Divide the mixture into equal amounts and shape each one into a small meatball.
4. Put them in the air fryer oven perforated pan and air fry for 7 minutes.
5. Transfer the meatballs to a baking dish and top with the tomato sauce and pasta sauce.
6. Set the dish into the air fryer oven and allow to air fry at 320ºF (160ºC) for 5 more minutes. Serve hot.

Teriyaki Pork and Mushroom Rolls

Prep time: 10 minutes | Cook time: 8 minutes | Serves 6

4 tablespoons brown sugar

4 tablespoons mirin

4 tablespoons soy sauce

1 teaspoon almond flour

2-inch ginger, chopped

6 (4-ounce / 113-g) pork belly slices

6 ounces (170 g) Enoki mushrooms

1. Mix the brown sugar, mirin, soy sauce, almond flour, and ginger together until brown sugar dissolves.
2. Take pork belly slices and wrap around a bundle of mushrooms. Brush each roll with teriyaki sauce. Chill for half an hour.
3. Set the temperature of the air fryer oven to 350ºF (177ºC) and add marinated pork rolls.
4. Air fry for 8 minutes. Flip the rolls halfway through.
5. Serve immediately.

Vietnamese Pork Chops

Prep time: 15 minutes | Cook time: 12 minutes | Serves 2

1 tablespoon chopped shallot

1 tablespoon chopped garlic

1 tablespoon fish sauce

3 tablespoons lemongrass

1 teaspoon soy sauce

1 tablespoon brown sugar

1 tablespoon olive oil

1 teaspoon ground black pepper

2 pork chops

1. Combine shallot, garlic, fish sauce, lemongrass, soy sauce, brown sugar, olive oil, and pepper in a bowl. Stir to mix well.
2. Put the pork chops in the bowl. Toss to coat well. Place the bowl in the refrigerator to marinate for 2 hours.
3. Set the temperature of the air fryer oven to 400ºF (204ºC). Press Start to begin preheating.
4. Remove the pork chops from the bowl and discard the marinade. Transfer the chops into the air fryer oven.
5. Air fry for 12 minutes or until lightly browned. Flip the pork chops halfway through the cooking time.
6. Remove the pork chops from the perforated pan and serve hot.

Poultry

Air Fried Chicken Fajitas

Prep time: 15 minutes | Cook time: 10 to 15 minutes | Serves 4

4 (5-ounce / 142-g) low-sodium boneless, skinless chicken breasts, cut into 4-by-½-inch strips

1 tablespoon freshly squeezed lemon juice

2 teaspoons olive oil

2 teaspoons chili powder

2 red bell peppers, sliced

4 low-sodium whole-wheat tortillas

$^{1}/_{3}$ cup nonfat sour cream

1 cup grape tomatoes, sliced

1. Set the temperature of the air fryer oven to 380ºF (193ºC). Press Start to begin preheating.
2. In a large bowl, mix the chicken, lemon juice, olive oil, and chili powder. Toss to coat.
3. Transfer the chicken to the air fryer oven perforated pan. Add the red bell peppers. Roast for 10 to 15 minutes, or until the chicken reaches an internal temperature of 165ºF (74ºC) on a meat thermometer.
4. Assemble the fajitas with the tortillas, chicken, bell peppers, sour cream, and tomatoes. Serve immediately.

Air Fried Naked Chicken Tenders

Prep time: 5 minutes | Cook time: 7 minutes | Serves 4

Seasoning:

1 teaspoon kosher salt

½ teaspoon garlic powder

½ teaspoon onion powder

½ teaspoon chili powder

¼ teaspoon sweet paprika

¼ teaspoon freshly ground black pepper

Chicken:

8 chicken breast tenders (1 pound / 454 g total)

2 tablespoons mayonnaise

1. Set the temperature of the air fryer oven to 375ºF (191ºC). Press Start to begin preheating.
2. For the seasoning: In a small bowl, combine the salt, garlic powder, onion powder, chili powder, paprika, and pepper.
3. For the chicken: Place the chicken in a medium bowl and add the mayonnaise. Mix well to coat all over, then sprinkle with the seasoning mix.
4. Working in batches, arrange a single layer of the chicken in the air fryer oven perforated pan. Air fry for 6 to 7 minutes, flipping halfway, until cooked through in the center. Serve immediately.

Almond-Crusted Chicken Nuggets

Prep time: 10 minutes | Cook time: 10 to 13 minutes | Serves 4

1 egg white

1 tablespoon freshly squeezed lemon juice

½ teaspoon dried basil

½ teaspoon ground paprika

1 pound (454 g) low-sodium boneless, skinless chicken breasts, cut into 1½-inch cubes

½ cup ground almonds

2 slices low-sodium whole-wheat bread, crumbled

1. Set the temperature of the air fryer oven to 400ºF (204ºC). Press Start to begin preheating.
2. In a shallow bowl, beat the egg white, lemon juice, basil, and paprika with a fork until foamy.
3. Add the chicken and stir to coat.
4. On a plate, mix the almonds and bread crumbs.
5. Toss the chicken cubes in the almond and bread crumb mixture until coated.

6. Bake the nuggets in the air fryer oven, in two batches, for 10 to 13 minutes, or until the chicken reaches an internal temperature of 165ºF (74ºC) on a meat thermometer. Serve immediately.

Apricot-Glazed Turkey Tenderloin

Prep time: 20 minutes | Cook time: 30 minutes | Serves 4

¼ cup sugar-free apricot preserves

½ tablespoon spicy brown mustard

1½ pounds (680 g) turkey breast tenderloin

Salt and freshly ground black pepper, to taste

Olive oil spray

1. Set the temperature of the air fryer oven to 370ºF (188ºC). Press Start to begin preheating. Spray the air fryer oven perforated pan lightly with olive oil spray.
2. In a small bowl, combine the apricot preserves and mustard to make a paste.
3. Season the turkey with salt and pepper. Spread the apricot paste all over the turkey.
4. Place the turkey in the air fryer oven perforated pan and lightly spray with olive oil spray.
5. Air fry for 15 minutes. Flip the turkey over and lightly spray with olive oil spray. Air fry until the internal temperature reaches at least 170ºF (77ºC), an additional 10 to 15 minutes.

6. Let the turkey rest for 10 minutes before slicing and serving.

Apricot-Glazed Chicken

Prep time: 5 minutes | Cook time: 12 minutes | Serves 2

2 tablespoons apricot preserves

½ teaspoon minced fresh thyme or ⅛ teaspoon dried

2 (8-ounce / 227-g) boneless, skinless chicken breasts, trimmed

1 teaspoon vegetable oil

Salt and pepper, to taste

1. Set the temperature of the air fryer oven to 400ºF (204ºC). Press Start to begin preheating.
2. Microwave apricot preserves and thyme in bowl until fluid, about 30 seconds; set aside. Pound chicken to uniform thickness as needed. Pat dry with paper towels, rub with oil, and season with salt and pepper.
3. Arrange breasts skin-side down in air fryer oven perforated pan, spaced evenly apart, alternating ends. Air fry the chicken for 4 minutes. Flip the chicken and brush skin side with apricot-thyme mixture. Air fry until chicken registers 160ºF (71ºC), 8 to 12 minutes more.
4. Transfer chicken to serving platter, tent loosely with aluminum foil, and let rest for 5 minutes. Serve.

Barbecue Chicken

Prep time: 10 minutes | Cook time: 18 to 20 minutes | Serves 4

$^{1}/_{3}$ cup no-salt-added tomato sauce

2 tablespoons low-sodium grainy mustard

2 tablespoons apple cider vinegar

1 tablespoon honey

2 garlic cloves, minced

1 jalapeño pepper, minced

3 tablespoons minced onion

4 (5-ounce / 142-g) low-sodium boneless, skinless chicken breasts

1. Set the temperature of the air fryer oven to 370ºF (188ºC). Press Start to begin preheating.
2. In a small bowl, stir together the tomato sauce, mustard, cider vinegar, honey, garlic, jalapeño, and onion.
3. Brush the chicken breasts with some sauce and air fry for 10 minutes.
4. Remove the air fryer oven perforated pan and turn the chicken; brush with more sauce. Air fry for 5 minutes more.
5. Remove the air fryer oven perforated pan and turn the chicken again; brush with more sauce. Air fry for 3 to 5 minutes more, or until the chicken reaches an internal temperature of 165ºF (74ºC) on a meat thermometer. Discard any remaining sauce. Serve immediately.

Barbecued Chicken with Creamy Coleslaw

Prep time: 10 minutes | Cook time: 20 minutes | Serves 2

3 cups shredded coleslaw mix

Salt and pepper

2 (12-ounce / 340-g) bone-in split chicken breasts, trimmed

1 teaspoon vegetable oil

2 tablespoons barbecue sauce, plus extra for serving

2 tablespoons mayonnaise

2 tablespoons sour cream

1 teaspoon distilled white vinegar, plus extra for seasoning

¼ teaspoon sugar

1. Set the temperature of the air fryer oven to 350ºF (177ºC). Press Start to begin preheating.

2. Toss coleslaw mix and ¼ teaspoon salt in a colander set over bowl. Let sit until wilted slightly, about 30 minutes. Rinse, drain, and dry well with a dish towel.

3. Meanwhile, pat chicken dry with paper towels, rub with oil, and season with salt and pepper. Arrange breasts skin-side down in air fryer oven perforated pan, spaced evenly apart, alternating ends. Bake for 10 minutes. Flip the breasts and brush skin side with

barbecue sauce. Return perforated pan to air fryer oven and bake until well browned and chicken registers 160ºF (71ºC), 10 to 15 minutes.

4. Transfer chicken to serving platter, tent loosely with aluminum foil, and let rest for 5 minutes. While chicken rests, whisk mayonnaise, sour cream, vinegar, sugar, and pinch pepper together in a large bowl. Stir in coleslaw mix and season with salt, pepper, and additional vinegar to taste. Serve chicken with coleslaw, passing extra barbecue sauce separately.

Blackened Chicken Breasts

Prep time: 10 minutes | Cook time: 20 minutes | Serves 4

1 large egg, beaten

¾ cup Blackened seasoning

2 whole boneless, skinless chicken breasts (about 1 pound / 454 g each), halved

Cooking spray

1. Set the temperature of the air fryer oven to 360ºF (182ºC). Press Start to begin preheating. Line the air fryer oven perforated pan with parchment paper.
2. Place the beaten egg in one shallow bowl and the Blackened seasoning in another shallow bowl.
3. One at a time, dip the chicken pieces in the beaten egg and the Blackened seasoning, coating thoroughly.
4. Place the chicken pieces on the parchment and spritz with cooking spray.
5. Air fry for 10 minutes. Flip the chicken, spritz with cooking spray, and air fry for 10 minutes more until the internal temperature reaches 165ºF (74ºC) and the

chicken is no longer pink inside. Let sit for 5 minutes before serving.

Buttermilk Paprika Chicken

Prep time: 7 minutes | Cook time: 17 to 23 minutes | Serves 4

4 (5-ounce / 142-g) low-sodium boneless, skinless chicken breasts, pounded to about ½ inch thick

½ cup buttermilk

½ cup all-purpose flour

2 tablespoons cornstarch

1 teaspoon dried thyme

1 teaspoon ground paprika

1 egg white

1 tablespoon olive oil

1. Set the temperature of the air fryer oven to 390ºF (199ºC). Press Start to begin preheating.
2. In a shallow bowl, mix the chicken and buttermilk. Let stand for 10 minutes.
3. Meanwhile, in another shallow bowl, mix the flour, cornstarch, thyme, and paprika.
4. In a small bowl, whisk the egg white and olive oil. Quickly stir this egg mixture into the flour mixture so the dry ingredients are evenly moistened.

5. Remove the chicken from the buttermilk and shake off any excess liquid. Dip each piece of chicken into the flour mixture to coat.
6. Air fry the chicken in the air fryer oven perforated pan for 17 to 23 minutes, or until the chicken reaches an internal temperature of 165ºF (74ºC) on a meat thermometer. Serve immediately.

Celery Chicken

Prep time: 10 minutes | Cook time: 15 minutes | Serves 4

½ cup soy sauce

2 tablespoons hoisin sauce

4 teaspoons minced garlic

1 teaspoon freshly ground black pepper

8 boneless, skinless chicken tenderloins

1 cup chopped celery

1 medium red bell pepper, diced

Cooking spray

1. Set the temperature of the air fryer oven to 375ºF (191ºC). Press Start to begin preheating. Spray the air fryer oven perforated pan lightly with olive oil spray.

2. In a large bowl, mix together the soy sauce, hoisin sauce, garlic, and black pepper to make a marinade. Add the chicken, celery, and bell pepper and toss to coat.

3. Shake the excess marinade off the chicken, place it and the vegetables in the air fryer oven perforated pan, and lightly spray with cooking spray. You may need to cook them in batches. Reserve the remaining marinade.

4. Air fry for 8 minutes. Turn the chicken over and brush with some of the remaining marinade. Air fry for an additional 5 to 7 minutes, or until the chicken reaches an internal temperature of at least 165ºF (74ºC). Serve.

Cheesy Chicken Tacos

Prep time: 10 minutes | Cook time: 12 to 16 minutes | Serves 2 to 4

1 teaspoon chili powder

½ teaspoon ground cumin

½ teaspoon garlic powder

Salt and pepper, to taste

Pinch cayenne pepper

1 pound (454 g) boneless, skinless chicken thighs, trimmed

1 teaspoon vegetable oil

1 tomato, cored and chopped

2 tablespoons finely chopped red onion

2 teaspoons minced jalapeño chile

1½ teaspoons lime juice

6 to 12 (6-inch) corn tortillas, warmed

1 cup shredded iceberg lettuce

3 ounces (85 g) Cheddar cheese, shredded (¾ cup)

1. Set the temperature of the air fryer oven to 400ºF (204ºC). Press Start to begin preheating.

2. Combine chili powder, cumin, garlic powder, ½ teaspoon salt, ¼ teaspoon pepper, and cayenne in bowl. Pat chicken dry with paper towels, rub with oil, and sprinkle evenly with spice mixture. Place chicken in air fryer oven perforated pan. Air fry until chicken registers 165ºF (74ºC), 12 to 16 minutes, flipping the chicken halfway through cooking.

3. Meanwhile, combine tomato, onion, jalapeño, and lime juice in a bowl; season with salt and pepper to taste and set aside until ready to serve.

4. Transfer chicken to a cutting board, let cool slightly, then shred into bite-size pieces using 2 forks. Serve chicken on warm tortillas, topped with salsa, lettuce, and Cheddar.

Chicken and Vegetable Fajitas

Prep time: 15 minutes | Cook time: 23 minutes | Serves 6

Chicken:

1 pound (454 g) boneless, skinless chicken thighs, cut crosswise into thirds

1 tablespoon vegetable oil

4½ teaspoons taco seasoning

Vegetables

1 cup sliced onion

1 cup sliced bell pepper

1 or 2 jalapeños, quartered lengthwise

1 tablespoon vegetable oil

½ teaspoon kosher salt

½ teaspoon ground cumin

For Serving:

Tortillas

Sour cream

Shredded cheese

Guacamole

Salsa

1. Set the temperature of the air fryer oven to 375ºF (191ºC). Press Start to begin preheating.

2. For the chicken: In a medium bowl, toss together the chicken, vegetable oil, and taco seasoning to coat.

3. For the vegetables: In a separate bowl, toss together the onion, bell pepper, jalapeño (s), vegetable oil, salt, and cumin to coat.

4. Place the chicken in the air fryer oven perforated pan. Air fry for 10 minutes. Add the vegetables to the perforated pan, toss everything together to blend the seasonings, and air fry for 13 minutes more. Use a meat thermometer to ensure the chicken has reached an internal temperature of 165ºF (74ºC).

5. Transfer the chicken and vegetables to a serving platter. Serve with tortillas and the desired fajita fixings.

Chicken Burgers with Ham and Cheese

Prep time: 12 minutes | Cook time: 13 to 16 minutes | Serves 4

$^{1}/_{3}$ cup soft bread crumbs

3 tablespoons milk

1 egg, beaten

½ teaspoon dried thyme

Pinch salt

Freshly ground black pepper, to taste

1¼ pounds (567 g) ground chicken

¼ cup finely chopped ham

$^{1}/_{3}$ cup grated Havarti cheese

Olive oil for misting

1. Set the temperature of the air fryer oven to 350ºF (177ºC). Press Start to begin preheating.

2. In a medium bowl, combine the bread crumbs, milk, egg, thyme, salt, and pepper. Add the chicken and mix gently but thoroughly with clean hands.

3. Form the chicken into eight thin patties and place on waxed paper.

4. Top four of the patties with the ham and cheese. Top with remaining four patties and gently press the edges together to seal, so the ham and cheese mixture is in the middle of the burger.

5. Place the burgers in the perforated pan and mist with olive oil. Bake for 13 to 16 minutes or until the chicken is thoroughly cooked to 165ºF (74ºC) as measured with a meat thermometer. Serve immediately.

Chicken Manchurian

Prep time: 10 minutes | Cook time: 20 minutes | Serves 2

1 pound (454 g) boneless, skinless chicken breasts, cut into 1-inch pieces

¼ cup ketchup

1 tablespoon tomato-based chili sauce, such as Heinz

1 tablespoon soy sauce

1 tablespoon rice vinegar

2 teaspoons vegetable oil

1 teaspoon hot sauce, such as Tabasco

½ teaspoon garlic powder

¼ teaspoon cayenne pepper

2 scallions, thinly sliced

Cooked white rice, for serving

1. Set the temperature of the air fryer oven to 350ºF (177ºC). Press Start to begin preheating.

2. In a bowl, combine the chicken, ketchup, chili sauce, soy sauce, vinegar, oil, hot sauce, garlic powder, cayenne, and three-quarters of the scallions and toss until evenly coated.

3. Scrape the chicken and sauce into a metal cake pan and place the pan in the air fryer oven. Bake until the chicken is cooked through and the sauce is reduced to a thick glaze, about 20 minutes, flipping the chicken pieces halfway through.
4. Remove the pan from the air fryer oven. Spoon the chicken and sauce over rice and top with the remaining scallions. Serve immediately.

Chicken Satay with Peanut Sauce

Prep time: 12 minutes | Cook time: 12 to 18 minutes | Serves 4

½ cup crunchy peanut butter

$^{1}/_{3}$ cup chicken broth

3 tablespoons low-sodium soy sauce

2 tablespoons lemon juice

2 cloves garlic, minced

2 tablespoons olive oil

1 teaspoon curry powder

1 pound (454 g) chicken tenders

1. Set the temperature of the air fryer oven to 390ºF (199ºC). Press Start to begin preheating.

2. In a medium bowl, combine the peanut butter, chicken broth, soy sauce, lemon juice, garlic, olive oil, and curry powder, and mix well with a wire whisk until smooth. Remove 2 tablespoons of this mixture to a small bowl. Put remaining sauce into a serving bowl and set aside.

3. Add the chicken tenders to the bowl with the 2 tablespoons sauce and stir to coat. Let stand for a few minutes to marinate, then run a bamboo skewer through each chicken tender lengthwise.

4. Put the chicken in the air fryer oven perforated pan and air fry in batches for 6 to 9 minutes or until the chicken reaches 165ºF (74ºC) on a meat thermometer. Serve the chicken with the reserved sauce.

Chicken with Pineapple and Peach

Prep time: 10 minutes | Cook time: 14 to 15 minutes | Serves 4

1 pound (454 g) low-sodium boneless, skinless chicken breasts, cut into 1-inch pieces

1 medium red onion, chopped

1 (8-ounce / 227-g) can pineapple chunks, drained, ¼ cup juice reserved

1 tablespoon peanut oil or safflower oil

1 peach, peeled, pitted, and cubed

1 tablespoon cornstarch

½ teaspoon ground ginger

¼ teaspoon ground allspice

Brown rice, cooked (optional)

1. Set the temperature of the air fryer oven to 380ºF (193ºC). Press Start to begin preheating.

2. In a medium metal bowl, mix the chicken, red onion, pineapple, and peanut oil. Bake in the air fryer oven for 9 minutes. Remove and stir.

3. Add the peach and return the bowl to the air fryer oven. Bake for 3 minutes more. Remove and stir again.

4. In a small bowl, whisk the reserved pineapple juice, the cornstarch, ginger, and allspice well. Add to the chicken mixture and stir to combine.

5. Bake for 2 to 3 minutes more, or until the chicken reaches an internal temperature of 165ºF (74ºC) on a meat thermometer and the sauce is slightly thickened.

6. Serve immediately over hot cooked brown rice, if desired.

Coconut Chicken Meatballs

Prep time: 10 minutes | Cook time: 14 minutes | Serves 4

1 pound (454 g) ground chicken

2 scallions, finely chopped

1 cup chopped fresh cilantro leaves

¼ cup unsweetened shredded coconut

1 tablespoon hoisin sauce

1 tablespoon soy sauce

2 teaspoons sriracha or other hot sauce

1 teaspoon toasted sesame oil

½ teaspoon kosher salt

1 teaspoon black pepper

1. Set the temperature of the air fryer oven to 350ºF (177ºC). Press Start to begin preheating.

2. In a large bowl, gently mix the chicken, scallions, cilantro, coconut, hoisin, soy sauce, sriracha, sesame oil, salt, and pepper until thoroughly combined (the mixture will be wet and sticky).

3. Place a sheet of parchment paper in the air fryer oven perforated pan. Using a small scoop or teaspoon, drop

rounds of the mixture in a single layer onto the parchment paper.

4. Air fry for 10 minutes, turning the meatballs halfway through the cooking time. Increase the temperature to 400ºF (204ºC) and air fry for 4 minutes more to brown the outsides of the meatballs. Use a meat thermometer to ensure the meatballs have reached an internal temperature of 165ºF (74ºC).
5. Transfer the meatballs to a serving platter. Repeat with any remaining chicken mixture. Serve.

Cranberry Curry Chicken

Prep time: 12 minutes | Cook time: 18 minutes | Serves 4

3 (5-ounce / 142-g) low-sodium boneless, skinless chicken breasts, cut into 1½-inch cubes

2 teaspoons olive oil

2 tablespoons cornstarch

1 tablespoon curry powder

1 tart apple, chopped

½ cup low-sodium chicken broth

$^{1}/_{3}$ cup dried cranberries

2 tablespoons freshly squeezed orange juice

Brown rice, cooked (optional)

1. Set the temperature of the air fryer oven to 380ºF (193ºC). Press Start to begin preheating.
2. In a medium bowl, mix the chicken and olive oil. Sprinkle with the cornstarch and curry powder. Toss to coat. Stir in the apple and transfer to a metal pan. Bake in the air fryer oven for 8 minutes, stirring once during cooking.
3. Add the chicken broth, cranberries, and orange juice. Bake for about 10 minutes more, or until the sauce is slightly thickened and the chicken reaches an internal temperature of 165ºF (74ºC) on a meat thermometer. Serve over hot cooked brown rice, if desired.

Crisp Chicken Wings

Prep time: 15 minutes | Cook time: 20 minutes | Serves 4

1 pound (454 g) chicken wings

3 tablespoons vegetable oil

½ cup all-purpose flour

½ teaspoon smoked paprika

½ teaspoon garlic powder

½ teaspoon kosher salt

1½ teaspoons freshly cracked black pepper

1. Set the temperature of the air fryer oven to 400ºF (204ºC). Press Start to begin preheating.

2. Place the chicken wings in a large bowl. Drizzle the vegetable oil over wings and toss to coat.

3. In a separate bowl, whisk together the flour, paprika, garlic powder, salt, and pepper until combined.

4. Dredge the wings in the flour mixture one at a time, coating them well, and place in the air fryer oven perforated pan. Air fry for 20 minutes, turning the wings halfway through the cooking time, until the breading is browned and crunchy.

5. Serve hot.

Crisp Paprika Chicken Drumsticks

Prep time: 5 minutes | Cook time: 22 minutes | Serves 2

2 teaspoons paprika

1 teaspoon packed brown sugar

1 teaspoon garlic powder

½ teaspoon dry mustard

½ teaspoon salt

Pinch pepper

4 (5-ounce / 142-g) chicken drumsticks, trimmed

1 teaspoon vegetable oil

1 scallion, green part only, sliced thin on bias

1. Set the temperature of the air fryer oven to 400ºF (204ºC). Press Start to begin preheating.

2. Combine paprika, sugar, garlic powder, mustard, salt, and pepper in a bowl. Pat drumsticks dry with paper towels. Using metal skewer, poke 10 to 15 holes in skin of each drumstick. Rub with oil and sprinkle evenly with spice mixture.

3. Arrange drumsticks in air fryer oven perforated pan, spaced evenly apart, alternating ends. Air fry until chicken is crisp and registers 195ºF (91ºC), 22 to 25 minutes, flipping the chicken halfway through cooking.

4. Transfer chicken to serving platter, tent loosely with aluminum foil, and let rest for 5 minutes. Sprinkle with scallion and serve.

CPSIA information can be obtained
at www.ICGtesting.com
Printed in the USA
LVHW081123160322
713512LV00009B/211

9 781804 503003